# *Advances in Hypnosis for Medicine, Dentistry, and Pain Prevention/Management*

## Donald C. Brown, M.D.

### Editor

**Crown House Publishing Limited**
www.crownhouse.co.uk
www.crownhousepublishing.com

First published by

Crown House Publishing Ltd
Crown Buildings, Bancyfelin, Carmarthen, Wales, SA33 5ND, UK
**www.crownhouse.co.uk**

and

Crown House Publishing Company LLC
6 Trowbridge Drive, Suite 5, Bethel, CT 06801-2858, USA
**www.crownhousepublishing.com**

**British Library Cataloguing-in-Publication Data**
A catalogue entry for this book is available
from the British Library.

**ISBN 978-184590120-2**

**LCCN 2008936802**

Printed and bound in the USA

The figures that appear in Chapter 3 (Figures 1–4 with accompanying instructions) are reprinted
with permission from *Trance and Treatment: Clinical Uses of Hypnosis*, Second Edition
(Copyright 2004). American Psychiatric Publishing, Inc.

*To Marlene E. Hunter, M.D.*

Marlene was the coordinating chair of the First Frontiers of Hypnosis held in Vancouver, British Columbia in 1986, which was hosted by the Hypnosis Society of British Columbia. And so Frontiers of Hypnosis, the first National Assembly of the Federation of Canadian Societies of Clinical Hypnosis, was born. The theme was on the innovation, the new and perhaps controversial, the cutting edge as it were, of research and inquiry into the clinical uses of hypnosis.

# Contents

# About the Contributors

A. Max Chaumette, MD, is a Diplomate of the American Boards of Anesthesiology and Medical Hypnosis. He has been a member of the faculty of several anesthesiology departments including Baylor College of Medicine and University of Chicago. Nowadays, he limits his practice to the use of hypnosis in the perioperative period and as an adjunct in the treatment of acute and chronic pain.

Gabor Filo, DDS, graduated in 1984 from the University of Toronto. He won Fellowship in the Academy of General Dentistry and has recently been admitted as an Honorary Fellow of the Pierre Fauchard Academy. An ardent proponent of dental hypnosis, he has, over the years, belonged to the major hypnosis societies, and has participated as faculty both locally and internationally. He is a Diplomate of the American Board of Hypnosis in Dentistry. His professional career includes solo and group practice, hospital dentistry, and an emphasis on the non-pharmacological treatment of dental anxiety and phobia. To further the latter, he has become an early adopter of hard and soft tissue laser dentistry, a subject area upon which he also lectures. Believing that one only improves one's milieu by joining in, he has extensive dental political experience as a Past President of the Hamilton Academy of Dentistry and through various positions at the Ontario Dental Association. Presently, he is the dental member-at-large for American Society of Clinical Hypnosis.

George A. Fraser MD, FRCPC, currently works as consultant psychiatrist to the Canadian Force's Operational Trauma and Stress Support Centre (Ottawa). He is a Fellow of the International Society for the Study of Trauma and Dissociation (ISSTD). He received the Pierre Janet Writing Award in 2003 from that society in 2003 for his publication of "Fraser's Dissociative Table Technique: Revised, Revisited." The latter is a strategy based on guided imagery and hypnosis for accessing and managing ego states in dissociative disorders. It is part of the core psychotherapy course provided by ISSTD.

Ashley A. Goodman, DDS, DABHD, DABFD, is a general dentist in private practice in San Diego, California, and an international educator in the fields of hypnosis and dentistry. He utilizes hypnosis, with a variety of induction techniques, on a regular basis for his patients and referrals. Dr. Goodman was the American Society of Clinical Hypnosis "Member At Large, Dentistry" representative, a member of the Board of Governors, Executive Board, numerous committees, and national workshop faculty, is a Certified and Approved Consultant, ASCH Fellow, and was presented with the Award of Merit 2001. He is also a past president, executive committee member, and a Fellow of his local San Diego Society of Clinical Hypnosis component. Additionally, he is a diplomat, board certified in hypnosis by the American Board of Hypnosis in Dentistry for which he serves as vice-president. Some of his dental affiliations include membership in Omicron Kappa Upsilon (National Dental Honor Society), American Dental Association, and San Diego County Dental Society, Academy of General Dentistry and Alpha Omega. He serves as an expert witness, technical investigator, and consultant in the field of dentistry and is a diplomat, board certified with the American Board of Forensic Dentistry/American College of Forensic Examiners.

Marlene E. Hunter, MD, FCFP(C) was a family physician for many years in West Vancouver until her work with trauma disorders overtook her practice. She is a Fellow and Certificant of the College of Family Physician of Canada and has been a Past President of the B.C. College of Family Physicians, the American Society of Clinical Hypnosis, the Canadian Society of Clinical Hypnosis (B.C. Division), and the International Society for Multiple Personality and Dissociation (now called the International Society for Trauma and Dissociation). She was Co-Chair of the Canadian Society for Trauma and Dissociation in its early years. Widely published, Dr. Hunter has written seven books as well as numerous contributions to other publications. Since the early 1980s, she has been a frequent presenter at international conferences and conventions and has taught this work in 19 countries. Since 2001, she has served as the Director of Labyrinth Victoria Centre for Dissociation (which she also owns) in Victoria, B.C.

Leora Kuttner, PhD, writes: "My focus for 30 years has been working with children to ease their distress in mind and body. This earned me a PhD in Clinical Psychology, a Professorship in Pediatrics at University of British Columbia & B.C. Children's Hospital and some unexpected honors. My first career in documentary film making at SABC-TV in South Africa wormed itself back. I needed to use that medium to show what children and teens could do with hypnosis and their natural talents. This led to the documentaries "No Fears, No Tears"(1986),"Children in Pain"(1989) "No Fears, No Tears – 13 Years Later" (1998) and "Making Every Moment Count" (2003). My book *A Child in Pain, How to Help What to Do*, which was written on sabbatical while training in acupuncture in Sri Lanka, will shortly be updated. With our two adult children in University, I'm curious to discover what is next!"

Bruce H. Lipton, PhD, bestselling author of *The Biology of Belief*, is a cellular biologist and former Associate Professor at the University of Wisconsin's School of Medicine. His pioneering research on cloned stem cells at Wisconsin presaged the revolutionary field of *epigenetics*, the new science of how environment and perception control genes. His later research at Stanford University's School of Medicine revealed the nature of the biochemical pathways that bridge the mind–body duality. His book, *The Biology of Belief: Unleashing the Power of Consciousness, Matter and Miracles* was released in 2005.

David A. Lovas, MD, obtained his science and medical degrees from Dalhousie University, before taking up his internship and residency training in Adult Psychiatry at Harvard Medical School, where he continues currently. Along with his clinical training, he is also involved in psychosomatic research, and was recently honored with the 2008–9 Dupont-Warren and Livingston Fellowships. Dr. Lovas also teaches Harvard medical students, and is an active committee member in several local and national medical professional organizations.

John G. L. Lovas, BSc, DDS, MSc, FRCD(C), obtained science and dental degrees from the University of Toronto, and specialty training in Oral Pathology at the University of Western Ontario. He recently retired from 25 years of part-time specialty private practice in Oral Medicine and Pathology, but remains a full-time Associate Professor at the Faculty of Dentistry, Dalhousie University, where he has taught Oral Pathology and Oral Medicine since 1983. He served as Chief Examiner in Oral Pathology and Oral Medicine for the Royal College of Dentists of Canada, and as President of the Canadian Academy of Oral Pathology. Dr. Lovas is currently in the process of formally introducing the concepts and practice of mindfulness into the undergraduate dental and dental hygiene curricula at the Dalhousie Faculty of Dentistry.

Jose R. Maldonado, MD, FAPM, FACFE, is Associate Professor of Psychiatry and Medicine; Chief, Medical and Forensic Psychiatry Section; Director, Medical Psychotherapy Clinic, Department of Psychiatry and Behavioral Sciences, Stanford University School of Medicine; and Medical Director, Psychosomatic Medicine Service, Stanford University Medical Center, Stanford, California.

David Spiegel, MD, is Willson Professor and Associate Chair of Psychiatry and Behavioral Sciences, Department of Psychiatry and Behavioral Sciences, Stanford University School of Medicine; and Medical Director, Stanford Center for Integrative Medicine, Stanford University Medical Center, Stanford, California.

James Straub, EdD, is a licensed psychologist/health service provider, has been a practicing therapist for more than 30 years. He is director and senior therapist of a multi-disciplinary counseling center, treatment director of a cognitive/behavioral partial hospitalization program and clinical assistant professor in the Department of Psychiatry, University of Missouri. He is the developer of Precision Cognitive Therapy and regularly lectures and provides workshops in the United States, Mexico, Canada, and France. He is an approved consultant with the American Society of Clinical Hypnosis, a Master Practitioner in NLP, Fellow at the American College of Forensic Examiners, Fellow at the International Academy of Eclectic Psychotherapy, and Diplomate of the American Board of Psychological Specialties in the area of trauma and PTSD.

Vicki W. Straub, PhD, MBA, is a licensed psychologist and member of the American Society of Clinical Hypnosis. She has a private practice background and more than 20 years as the coordinator of the behavioral science/behavioral medicine program in the Family Medicine Residency Program at the University of Missouri. Her training includes clinical hypnosis, traumatology, Neurolinguistic Programming, cognitive therapy, Adlerian therapy, and Imago Therapy. She has lectured and presented workshops in the United States, Canada, Mexico, and France. She also works as a consultant in the medical and business community as a trainer in team building, stress management, negotiation/mediation, and executive coaching.

# Acknowledgments

I deeply appreciate the support and generosity of my colleagues who have contributed to this book. They have spent many hours rewriting the plenary and workshop presentations that comprise its chapters; their expertise greatly enriches the value of this book as a reliable resource.

My gratitude is also extended to the following people:

- Eleanore, my wife, for her patience, support, and endurance of my absences.

- Kelly Underwood for her many hours of secretarial assistance in organizing the 6th Frontiers of Hypnosis and early work on the book chapters, and Angela Faulkner, who has served as our typist for this last year.

- The librarians at Dalhousie Kellogg Health Sciences Library, who were so helpful during literature searches.

- Crown House Publishing, especially Mark Tracten, President, for his suggestion, encouragement, and support in producing this book. And to Suzi Tucker, our editor, who was most helpful in improving the clarity and flow of a number of chapters as we prepared this manuscript to see the light of day.

# Foreword

I have known Dr. Donald Brown for over 15 years. We first met at the Frontiers of Hypnosis National Assembly in Vancouver in 1992 and since then we have met at various national and international conferences in clinical hypnosis. More recently I invited Dr. Brown to write an evidence-based review paper on obstetrics, particularly on the effectiveness of hypnosis in labor and delivery for the *International Journal of Clinical and Experimental Hypnosis* (2007). Dr. Brown has been involved in the scientific study, teaching and application of hypnosis since he started family practice in the 1959. After joining the Faculty of Medicine at Dalhousie Medical School, he taught clinical hypnosis to graduate and undergraduate medical students and conducted seminars and training for psychotherapists, physicians and other health professionals. His recent activities also include organizing and coordinating various regional, national and international conferences in hypnosis. Despite a busy schedule, he also has managed to conduct research and continue producing papers on clinical hypnosis. All of this is to say that Dr. Brown has the right credentials for editing a book on *Advances in Hypnosis for Medicine, Dentistry, and Pain Prevention/Management*, which, as the title suggests, focuses on applying hypnosis to the management of medical and dental conditions.

The idea for the book and the majority of the chapters contained here originated from the 6th Frontiers of Hypnosis National Assembly, October 9–12, 2003, in Halifax, Nova Scotia, Canada, which was coordinated by Dr. Brown. Requested by the publisher to produce a book on clinical hypnosis applied to medicine and dentistry, Dr. Brown had to consider the wealth of material from the conference, presented by both world-renowned and relatively unknown professionals, reflecting a range of disciplines, and then create a balanced and healthy product. Dr. Brown succeeded admirably with this difficult task by sticking to Hippocrates's proposition that "Nothing should be omitted in an art which interests the whole world, one which may be beneficial to suffering humanity and which does not risk life or comfort." Hypnotherapy is an art and there is abundant evidence that hypnosis alleviates suffering and improves human well-being. Hence, as early as 1955, the British Medical Association accepted hypnosis as a legitimate therapy in medical practice. This was followed by the American Medical Association in 1958. Similarly, in 1961, the American Psychiatric Association accepted hypnosis as a specialized psychiatric procedure. Even more significantly, in 1965 the Canadian Medical Association accepted hypnosis in medical practice and medical school curricula. Despite the official endorsement of clinical hypnosis, the acceptance of hypnosis in the medical communities has been controversial. It is hoped that this book will reduce some of these uncertainties.

*Advances in Hypnosis for Medicine, Dentistry, and Pain Prevention/Management* consists primarily of hypnotherapy techniques applied to medicine and dentistry. The chapters are organized in three sections – medical hypnosis, dental hypnosis, and pain management. The medical hypnosis section includes five chapters by Spiegel, Maldonado, Lipton, Fraser and Hunter. In the opening chapter, Spiegel and Maldonado remark that the focus of modern medicine is on developing and administering biotechnological treatments, rather than helping patients through their illness. They believe hypnosis provides a method for addressing this unmet need by helping patients utilize their focused attention to reduce anxiety, pain, maladaptive habits and psychosomatic symptoms. They argue that hypnosis can help patients alter their experience of medical procedures and they cite research by Elvira Lang and her colleagues to support their argument. Lang and her colleagues demonstrated that patients undergoing interventional radiological procedures using arterial access used half the pain medication, felt less pain, had fewer complications, experienced faster recovery afterward and got through in an average of 17 minutes less time, which resulted in a cost saving of $338 per procedure.

Lipton explores how hypnosis can override genetic programming and how belief can affect treatment outcome. He examines the *new biology* of how the physical body can be affected by the immaterial mind. He reviews the influence of energy on the brain and on the body's physiology and argues that harnessing the power of the mind can be more effective than drugs in the management of a variety of medical and psychological disorders. He provides insight into how the body's mind–body pathways work to produce physical improvement. He highlights the findings that both perception and environment directly controls the activity of the genes. Lipton's hypothesis that beliefs control biology is grounded in studies of cloned endothelial cells that line the blood vessels. He believes hypnotherapy facilitates by altering the patient's perception of the patient's environment and thus thought alters biological expression.

Spiegel and Fraser discuss the advantages of using formal measures of hypnotic responsivity, especially the Hypnotic Induction Profile (HIP), which takes 6 to 10 minutes to administer. Marlene Hunter describes the usefulness of mind–body communication in hypnotherapy. She focuses particularly on how to utilize mind–body communication with patients with psychosomatic disorders. She describes various hypnotherapeutic techniques for modifying psychosomatic behaviors and adopting more adaptive behaviors. Although the use hypnotic suggestibility measures in clinical practice is hotly debated, from an empirical perspective it is advisable to measure hypnotic responsivity as an independent measure.

Section II is dedicated to dental hypnosis. John and David Lovas describe the uniqueness of dental practice and the need for effective and rapid hypnotic techniques. Their chapter deals with identifying and treating dental anxiety with rapid hypnotic relaxation. Nearly one half the people in the United States express some fear toward dentistry. This fear ranges from mild apprehension to paralyzing anxieties. Approximately 30 million of these people have a fear so great that they are termed phobic and avoid dental care completely. Numerous edentulous patients never had dentures made or have dentures they never wear because of overt gag responses. An overt or excessive gag reflex is usually a learned or conditional response, and thus, it can be unlearned. The chapter by Filo is thought-provoking and innovative. He provides validation for utilizing hypnosis in high-tech dentistry. He argues that although technological advances are very important in dental medicine, they are not sufficient. He describes how to integrate hypnosis in dental practice, and separates hypnosis into two broad overlapping categories: psychological and physiological applications. In the final chapter of this section, Goodman and Brown deal with pain, anxiety and gagging in adults and children.

Pain management is the subject of Section III. Dr. Chaumette describes the use of hypnosis in perioperative procedures, with acute and chronic pain, and as a complement during pregnancy, labor and delivery. James and Vicki Straub deal with specific traumatic memories such as motor vehicle accidents or childhood physical or sexual abuse that may be related to persistent pain or triggered during procedures. Dr. Kuttner examines how hypnosis can be applied as a therapeutic intervention across the wide age range of ages from young children to late teens (3–19 years) and considers changes required in hypnotic process when used at different developmental stages. She offers therapeutic recommendations on how to use hypnosis with common pediatric problems such as anxiety, sleep problems, acute pain, recurrent pain and chronic pain.

Dr. Brown ends the section with an in-depth review of the benefits and effectiveness of hypnosis in obstetrics and in labor and delivery. He demonstrates that the application of hypnosis in these areas significantly reduces the necessity of analgesics and anesthesia and shortens stage one and stage two labor.

This book provides a rich source of information for the use of hypnosis in medicine and dentistry. This is not a cookbook but a comprehensive source of reference.

Assen Alladin, Ph.D., R.Psych.
Clinical Psychologist
Adjunct Associate Professor
Past President of Canadian Federation of Clinical Hypnosis – Alberta Society
Education Chair of Canadian Federation of Clinical Hypnosis

Author of *Handbook of Cognitive Hypnotherapy for Depression: An Evidence-Based Approach* (2007), *Hypnotherapy Explained* (2008), *Cognitive Hypnotherapy: An Integrated Approach to the Treatment of Emotional Disorders* (2008)

# *Preface*

The most important five minutes of life are the first five minutes after birth. How soon we breathe after being born may determine how quick we are the rest of our lives.

I started doing hypnosis in my family practice after a patient asked me to show her how to use hypnosis for her second labor and delivery. She'd had a prolonged and difficult delivery the first time around, and she did not want to go through the experience again. She did so well with the second birth that she said she would use hypnosis again if she decided to have any more children.

That was more than 44 years ago, and that early lesson stayed with me throughout my career. There were years when I have delivered more than 100 babies, and over half of my obstetrical patients chose to use hypnosis for labor and delivery. As a busy practitioner, their choice saved me a great deal of time because labors were shorter, with fewer examinations needed, and few medications prescribed. Over 50 percent of my patients required nothing more than hypnosis – that is, no anesthetics or analgesics.

That is a little of my specific experience, but the inspiration for this book came out of the many profound perspectives presented at the 6th Frontiers of Hypnosis Assembly in Halifax, Nova Scotia in 2003. The bulk of the present material was culled from 11 of the groundbreaking workshops that were presented there. All the material has been rewritten and updated by the authors.

The goal of the book is to feature the work of those who are expert in the use of hypnosis across a spectrum of settings and applications so that clinicians who wish to use it – or who already do – have access to the most in-depth information available on the biology of hypnosis as it pertains to medicine, dentistry, and pain prevention and management.

Because I believe that hypnosis is a much underutilized modality, this book has several purposes: to encourage more clinicians to start using hypnosis in their practices; to offer solid information on the biology of hypnosis and advances of clinical uses of hypnosis and self-hypnosis; and to present an overview of the big picture – the breadth and depth of clinical hypnosis for those who use it in their practices. A very useful feature of this book is the reference sections at the end of each chapter for those who wish to find further information on the topic. Additional general hypnosis books are suggested in the reference section at the end of Chapter 8.

Under Medical Hypnosis you will find chapters on the biology of hypnosis, mind–body communication, and psychosomatic medicine, among others. Under Dental Hypnosis, there are discussions of the practical management of pre-op anxiety, validating the use of hypnosis, and dealing with pain and anxiety in adults and children. In the section on Pain Prevention and Management, the authors address the use of hypnosis in anesthesiology, resolving traumatic and key decision memories in the treatment of pain and treating pain, anxiety, and sleep disorders in children and adolescents.

The final chapter of the book is a research report that will provide readers with a current view on findings that clarify the significance of the central role of hypnosis in obstetrics, labor, and delivery, including the use of self-hypnosis to prevent pain and premature childbirth. Prenatal hypnosis has been shown to positively affect the health of the newborn infant on a number of levels. This chapter emphasizes the importance of clinicians doing hypnosis research in their practices and publishing their findings.

Every chapter in this book focuses on an important application for the use of hypnosis, beginning at the beginning…the most important five minutes of life are the first five minutes after being born.

# Part I
# *Medical Hypnosis*

# Chapter 1

# *Hypnosis in Medicine*

*David Spiegel and Jose Maldonado*

Hypnosis, the oldest Western form of psychotherapy (Ellenberger, 1970), is also one of the newest means of helping people cope with the rigors of high-tech medicine. The rapid technological advances in modern medicine and its successes have only increased the number of people living with chronic and serious illness. Furthermore, the growing emphasis in medicine on pharmacological treatments, minimally invasive surgery, and advanced imaging techniques has created more need for techniques that help people through medical procedures without general anesthesia. By and large doctors have concentrated on developing and administering the treatments, rather than on helping patients through them. Almost half of North Americans utilize some form of complementary or integrative medical technique (Eisenberg, Davis et al., 1998). This growing and seemingly paradoxical interest in integrative medicine can be understood as a response to this problem – the human need behind the biotechnological direction of medicine. In addition, the growth of managed care and insurance-dominated medicine has disrupted doctor–patient relationships by mandating frequent changes in medical care and constraining the time doctors can spend with patients. Hypnosis can help medicine address some of these challenges, utilizing a patient's ability to focus attention to help with many medically related problems – anxiety, pain, habit control, and psychosomatic disorders.

## *Hypnosis*

Hypnosis is a state of aroused, attentive, focused concentration with a relative suspension of peripheral awareness (Spiegel & Spiegel, 2004). It is comprised of three main components: absorption, dissociation, and suggestibility. It is a state that can be entered in a matter of seconds, if the patient has the requisite hypnotizability. The ability to experience hypnosis is a stable and measurable trait. The Hypnotic Induction Profile (Spiegel & Spiegel, 2004) was developed for the clinical setting, takes five minutes to administer, and provides reliable data about a patient's hypnotizability, while teaching the patient how to commence utilizing self-hypnosis. This approach takes the onus off of the clinician to "get the patient into a trance," and off of patients to comply rather than explore their hypnotic ability. The therapist is free to focus on evaluating the patient's ability to enter the state, rather than on getting the person into the state. Further, such a standardized testing induction permits an important deduction regarding the hypnotic capacity of the subject. The restricted range of input from the therapist using the test protocol maximizes the information provided by variations in subjects' responses. After discussing the results of the testing with the subject, both can proceed knowledgeably, choosing to use hypnosis or other techniques in the service of an agreed-upon treatment goal.

Hypnotizability testing provides objective data about the patient's ability to respond to treatment employing hypnosis. If the patient is a highly hypnotizable individual, he or she can be rationally encouraged to proceed with the use of hypnosis. Non-hypnotizable individuals can be offered an alternative approach that is likely to be more efficacious, such as relaxation techniques, biofeedback, or medication.

## *Measuring Hypnotizability*

The Hypnotic Induction Profile (HIP) is a useful clinical screening test for hypnotic capacity. It consists of a number of simple instructions that allow for the measurement of patients' natural ability to tap into and use their hypnotic capacity. It begins with a simple and quick induction, counting from one to three, accompanied by the eye roll, which involves instructed upward gaze and lowering of the eyelids. The dissociation between upward gaze and lowering of the eyelid can be scored, providing the therapist with an initial prediction of the subject's hypnotic capacity. The eye roll is then followed by a series of instructions to briefly influence the subject's behavior during and shortly after the test (post-hypnotic suggestions). The HIP allows the therapist to rate the subject on five items assessing cognitive and behavioral aspects of the single continuous but brief hypnotic experience elicited during the test. The items are: (1) their ability to experience a sense of *dissociation* of the left hand from the rest of the body; (2) *hand levitation*, or the movement of the hand, floating back up in the air after being pulled down; (3) a sense of *involuntariness or unconscious compliance* while elevating the hand; (4) response to the *cut-off* signal ending the hypnotic experience; and (5) a *sensory alteration* in the hand or elsewhere in the body.

Scores on the HIP are significantly but moderately correlated with those on the Stanford Scales (Orne, Hilgard et al., 1979; Frischholz, Tryon et al., 1980).

# *Hypnosis in Medical Procedures*

Because of the power of hypnosis to enhance focus of attention and trigger dissociation, it can be highly effective in helping patients to alter their experience of medical procedures. Useful techniques include the following:

1.  *Float.* Hypnotic affiliation with a somatic metaphor that connotes but does not directly instruct relaxation can help reduce muscle tension and a sense of struggle during the procedure: "Imagine that you are floating in a bath, a lake, a hot tub, or just floating in space."

2.  *Pleasant scene.* This involves instructing patients to imagine that they are somewhere else that they find pleasant and safe. This allows them to dissociate their mental preoccupation from their immediate medical surroundings, thereby reducing secondary anxiety.

3.  *Pain reduction.* Patients can be taught to alter perception in any part of their body where they are experiencing discomfort: "Imagine a sense of tingling numbness, coolness, warmth, lightness or heaviness. These sensations will filter the hurt out of the pain." Less hypnotizable patients can be taught to focus on sensations in another unaffected part of their body, for example rubbing their fingertips together.

Such simple instructions have been found to be highly effective in reducing pain, anxiety, complications of procedures, and even in reducing the time required for the procedures themselves. For example, in one large randomized trial, Lang and colleagues (Lang, Benotsch et al., 2000) found that patients undergoing interventional radiological procedures using arterial access required half the pain medication, felt less pain, had fewer complications, experienced faster recovery afterward, and got through in an average of 17 minutes less time. Despite the cost of employing a trained professional to teach hypnosis, this resulted in an overall saving of $338 per procedure (Lang & Rosen, 2002).

We have found similar results for children undergoing bladder catherization. Children facing voiding cystourethrograms were taught how to use self-hypnosis, with reinforcement from a parent who guided the exercise. They learned to imagine they were at a playground, amusement park, or a friend's house playing. They had less distress, the technicians reported that the catherization was easier, and the approach saved an average of 18 minutes per procedure (a long 18 minutes for a child in distress). (Butler, Symons et al., 2005).

Indeed, hypnosis is especially effective in comforting children who are in pain. Several good studies have shown greater efficacy than placebo attention control in randomized trials. Their imaginative capacities are so intense that separate relaxation exercises are usually unnecessary. Children naturally relax when they utilize their imagination, and tend to be more hypnotizable than adults (Gardner & Olness, 1981; Kuttner, 1988; Kuttner, 1989; Kuttner, 1993). Earlier studies have demonstrated that hypnotic analgesia is highly effective in the medical setting with children (Zeltzer & LeBaron, 1982; Zeltzer, LeBaron et al., 1984).

## Pain Control

James Esdaile (1846), a Scottish surgeon working in India, reported 80% surgical anesthesia for amputations using hypnosis. He also reported a lower mortality rate (5%) with his procedures than those in Great Britain (40%), probably due to the high risks of anesthesia at that time. However, he later withdrew his findings after being severely censured by his colleagues.

Despite the organic factors causing pain, it is clear that psychological factors are major variables in the intensity of the pain experience. Ninety years after Esdaile, at the Massachusetts General Hospital, Beecher (1956) demonstrated that the intensity of pain was directly associated with its meaning. For example, to the extent that pain represented an existential threat and the possibility of future disability, it was more intense than it was among a group of combat soldiers to whom the pain of injury meant that they were likely to get out of combat alive (Kardiner & Spiegel, 1947).

Hypnosis can facilitate an alteration in the subjective experience of pain (Brose & Spiegel, 1992). Several techniques can be used to achieve this goal. Most techniques involve the production of physical relaxation coupled with visual or somatic imagery that provides a substitute focus of attention for the painful sensation. The specific technique employed may depend on the degree of hypnotic ability of the subject. For example, patients can be taught to develop a comfortable floating sensation on the affected body part. Highly hypnotizable individuals may simply imagine a shot of Novocain in the affected area, producing a sense of tingling numbness similar to that experienced in previous dental work. Other patients may prefer to move the pain to another part of their body, or to dissociate the affected part from the rest of the body. As an extreme form of hypnotically induced, controlled dissociation, some patients may imagine themselves floating above their own body, creating distance between themselves and the painful sensation or experience. To some more moderately hypnotizable patients it may be easier to focus on a change in temperature, either warmth or coolness. A sensation of warmth might be elicited while imagining they are floating in a warm bath or applying a heating pad to a given area of the body. A cooling sensation can be elicited by imagining that the afflicted extremity is immersed in an ice-cold mountain stream or in a bucket of ice chips. Temperature metaphors are extraordinarily effective. This may be related to the fact that pain and temperature fibers run together in the lateral spinothalamic tract.

All the possible images or metaphors employed for pain control use certain general principles. The first is that the hypnotically controlled image may serve to "filter the hurt out of the pain." The patients also learn to transform the pain experience. They acknowledge that it exists (the pain) but that there is a distinction between the signal itself and the discomfort the signal causes. The hypnotic experience that they create and control helps them transform the signal into one that is less uncomfortable. So patients expand their perceptual options by having them change from an experience in which either the pain is there or it is not, to one in which they see a third option, in which the pain is there but transformed by the presence of such competing sensations as tingling, numbness, warmth, or coolness. Finally, patients are taught not to fight the pain. Fighting pain only enhances it by focusing attention on it, increasing related anxiety and depression, and intensifying physical tension, which can literally put traction on painful parts of the body and increase the pain signals generated peripherally.

For patients undergoing painful procedures, such as chemotherapy or bone marrow aspirations, the main focus is on the hypnotic imagery per se rather than on relaxation. This works especially well with children since they are so highly hypnotizable and easily absorbed in images. Patients may be guided through the experience while the procedure is being performed or a given scenario is suggested and later they revisit the experience hypnotically while the procedure is underway. This enables patients to restructure their experience of what is going on and dissociate themselves psychologically from pain and fear of the procedure.

Hypnotic analgesia works. A report from the Office of Technology Assessment (NIH Technology, 1996) concluded that hypnosis is a proven technique for reducing pain. Furthermore, in a randomized prospective study, a combination of hypnosis and group psychotherapy was shown to result in a 50% reduction in pain among metastatic breast cancer patients (Spiegel & Bloom, 1983), and there was a corresponding reduction in mood disturbance (Spiegel, Bloom et al., 1981). Hypnotic analgesia has also been shown to be more potent than either placebo analgesia (McGlashan, Evans et al., 1969) or acupuncture analgesia (Knox & Shum, 1977), although there is a correlation between hypnotizability and responsiveness to acupuncture (Katz, Kao et al., 1974). Thus, hypnotic mechanisms of pain control may be mobilized by other treatment techniques, but the explicit use of hypnosis with hypnotizable patients has proved to be more a powerful means of controlling pain.

Hypnotic analgesia seems to work via three mechanisms: physical relaxation, sensory alteration, and a change in the meaning of the pain. Patients in pain tend to splint the painful area instinctively, and yet this enhanced muscle tension around a painful area often increases pain. Most patients find that they can enhance their physical repose by focusing on a variety of images that connote physical relaxation such as a sense of floating. Second, and probably more important, since hypnosis involves an intensification and narrowing of the focus of attention, it allows individuals to alter their perception of the pain itself, placing pain at the periphery of their awareness by replacing it with some competing metaphor or sensation at the center of their attention. Thus, by focusing on a memory of dental anesthesia and spreading that numbness to the affected area, making the area warmer or cooler, substituting a sense of tingling or lightness, or focusing on sensation in some non-painful part of the body, hypnotized individuals can diminish the amount of pain they experience. Third, they can learn to alter the importance of the pain signals, reducing response to them. Recent research utilizing positron emission tomography has shown that hypnotic instructions to alter pain intensity reduce blood flow in somatosensory cortex, while instructions to find that the pain is less troublesome result in reduction of blood flow in the anterior cingulate gyrus (Rainville, Duncan et al., 1997; Rainville, Carrier et al., 1999; Rainville, Bushnell et al., 2001; Rainville, Hofbauer et al., 2002).

That hypnotic analgesia is not merely social compliance but involves neurophysiological changes in information processing has been shown also by studies of cortical event-related potential studies in which highly hypnotizable individuals could diminish the $P_{100}$ and $P_{300}$ components of their event-related response to a somatosensory stimulus by focusing on a hallucinated image which would block their perception of the stimulus (Spiegel, Bierre et al., 1989; DePascalis, 1999) There is also evidence using PET of reversible changes in processing of visual color stimuli consistent with the direction of change (Kosslyn, Thompson et al., 2000). Thus when hypnotized to see color in a black and white grid, subjects demonstrated increased blood flow in the portion of the occipital cortex that processes color vision, while an instruction to drain color from a color image decreased blood flow in this region. Hypnotic sensory alteration changes actual perceptual processes, not just the reaction to them.

## *Psychosomatic Disorders*

Most patients with high hypnotizability also have an unusual capacity for psychological control over somatic function. This is witnessed in cases of psychosomatic disorders, as well as in cases of conversion reactions. Consequently, hypnotic control over somatic function can be a two-edged sword. It is possible that these individuals have turned their capacity for somatic control against themselves. If this is true, then it makes sense that hypnosis be used in the control and treatment of these symptoms. For example, in 1975 Andreychuk and Skriver (Andreychuk & Skriver, 1975) found that high hypnotizability was both a good predictor of pretreatment symptom severity, as well as of treatment response for migraine headache patients. That is, more highly hypnotizable individuals complained of more severe migraine symptoms prior to treatment, but responded better to intervention.

When considered in cases of psychosomatic illnesses hypnosis is useful in both diagnosis and the treatment. By using hypnosis with these patients the therapist may assist in diagnosing the symptoms as psychosomatic. Under hypnosis many of the symptoms may improve or completely reverse. It is important though not to "force a cure" in any patient, but rather to allow the patient to improve at a pace that feels comfortable, or to give up the symptom when ready. This allows patients to feel in control, not only of the treatment and recovery process, but to reclaim their sense of control over their body. Some patients obtain insight into what is happening to their bodies due to the ability to explore the meaning and etiology of the symptoms hypnotically. In most instances it is better if hypnosis is used as an adjuvant to any other medical treatment, including physical rehabilitation or any other treatment modality typically used in the treatment of the "real illness."

Another goal of hypnosis is to allow the patient to understand the effects of emotional stress on their body, sometimes by demonstrating to the patient, under hypnosis, their ability to intensify or reduce symptoms for which they now seek help. Afterwards they are helped to retrain their minds in order to control their response.

Hypnosis can be invaluable in the treatment of a number of psychosomatic conditions. Disorders affecting the gastro-intestinal (GI) system are among those conditions in which studies demonstrated a dramatic response. In cases of ulcerative colitis and regional enteritis, patients have found it helpful to imagine in trance something soothing in their gut. This gives them a sense of control over a symptom that renders them feeling especially helpless, thereby diminishing the cycle of reactive anxiety. Actually, Whorwell and colleagues (Whorwell, Prior et al., 1984; Whorwell, Prior et al., 1987; Colgan, Faragher et al., 1988; Calvert, Houghton et al., 2002) demonstrated how patients with irritable bowel syndrome who were treated with hypnosis reported significant improvement in pain, abdominal distention, and diarrhea, as well as emotional well-being, compared to a control group. Follow-up of these patients showed continued remission of the symptoms.

In studies related to peptic ulcer disease (PUD), Klein and Spiegel (1989) observed significant hypnotic control of gastric acid secretion among highly hypnotizable subjects. They were initially instructed (under hypnosis) to consume an imaginary meal. This was accompanied by a raise in basal acid output of 89%. This was followed by another study in which subjects were instructed to use hypnosis to experience deep relaxation. These patients experienced a significant drop in basal acid output of 39%. In a third trial, subjects were given an injection of pentagastrin, in order to stimulate maximal parietal cell output. Even with this chemical stimulus, there was a significant 11% reduction in peak acid output when hypnosis was used. Finally, an independent study by Colgan, Faragher, & Whorwell (1988) randomly assigned a group of peptic ulcer disease patients to either hypnosis or no treatment (control) after an initial treatment with ranitidine. The results: 100% of the patients in the control group relapsed, compared to only 53% of those in the hypnosis group.

Several studies have proven the efficacy of hypnosis in the treatment of other psychosomatic conditions including warts (Ewin, 1992; Spanos, Stenstrom et al., 1988); bronchial asthma (Aronof, Aronoff et al., 1975; Ewer & Stewart, 1986; Kohen, Olness et al., 1984; Morrison, 1988), and cardiovascular problems, such as angina pectoris (Greenleaf, Fisher et al., 1992; Weinstein & Au, 1991).

The above examples further emphasize the fact that high hypnotizability is a two-edged sword. It may increase or decrease a given physiological parameter, depending on the mental content during the hypnotic state. Unfortunately, many patients unconsciously use it to their detriment. The goal of treatment then is to train them on how to master their hypnotic capacity and use it to normalize and regulate bodily functions.

# *Applications of Hypnosis in Habit Control*

## *Smoking Cessation*

There are a number of studies that demonstrate the efficacy of hypnosis as a tool to facilitate control of smoking habits. These studies show success rates in cigarette abstinence after treatment with hypnosis ranging from 13–64%. In these studies abstinence is defined as no smoking during a follow-up time of at least six months (Schwartz, 1987). H. Spiegel (Spiegel, 1970) developed a single-session approach for smoking cessation which is widely used (Schwartz, 1987). His results have been replicated and shown to produce outcomes of 20–35% long-term complete abstinence (Berkowitz, Ross-Townsend et al., 1979; Barabasz, Baer et al., 1986; Frank, Umlauf et al., 1986; Spiegel, 1970; Spiegel & Spiegel, 1987). Others have reported abstinence rates as high as 40% at six months (Hyman, Stanley et al., 1986; Williams & Hall, 1988). These numbers are better than the rates of unassisted quitting (Gritz & Bloom, 1987). Studies have also shown that higher hypnotizability predicts better outcome (Spiegel & Spiegel, 1987; Barabasz, Baer et al., 1986; Spiegel, Frischholz et al., 1993).

There are several mechanisms by which hypnosis may contribute to the above success in smoking cessation. The ritualistic process of the hypnotic exercise may provide a kind of substitute physical relaxation for the "breathing exercise" that accompanies the act of smoking; the positive affirmations in self-hypnosis provide positive reinforcement for behavior change and promote positive self image; its use enhances self-observation and self-monitoring; and finally it facilitates cognitive restructuring of the smoking habit.

The single session method developed by H. Spiegel (Spiegel, 1970) emphasizes teaching patients self-hypnosis rather than having multiple sessions with a therapist. It uses a strategy that is intrinsically self-reinforcing and meaningful to the patient. It can be practiced whenever the urge to smoke comes upon the patient. This method of cognitive restructuring involves emphasizing that the act of smoking is destructive to the patient's body and thereby limits what the patient can do with his or her life; it shortens lifespan, and deteriorates quality of life. Hypnosis is used to emphasize the patient's commitment to protect the body from the poison of cigarettes. This approach gives the patient the ability to examine priorities and to balance the urge to smoke against the urge to protect his or her body from damage. At the end the patient has the option to choose between what he or she is for, rather than what he or she is against (Spiegel, 1970).

In summary, there is no evidence that treatments employing hypnosis are more effective than other interventions for smoking. Nevertheless, they may be more efficient because such treatments enable patients to employ a self-administered treatment strategy (self-hypnosis) to reinforce a more adaptive cognitive restructuring, while providing them with an exercise in physical relaxation (Spiegel & Spiegel, 2004).

## Weight Control

Hypnosis, when employed, is usually utilized as an adjunct to a comprehensive dietary and exercise control program for weight reduction and management. Similar to the use of self-hypnosis in the control of smoking, in dietary control the purpose is to restructure patients' experience with overeating. Patients are asked to examine their excess food intake and to pay attention to the damaging effects to their body. This then translates into an exercise about learning to eat with respect for one's body. As with smoking control, the emphasis is on what the patient is for, rather than against.

An important component of such an approach is teaching the patient to use self-hypnosis training to control the urge to overeat. This is better accomplished by preparing a list of food that reflects eating with respect and then comparing a given urge with the list. If the desired food is on the list, the patient is encouraged to eat it like a gourmet, focusing intently on all aspects of the eating experience and enjoying it. If the food is not on the list, the patient is asked to recognize the desire, rather than fight the urge. Then the patient is encouraged to use self-hypnosis to compare this urge with his or her overall commitment to protect and treat his or her body with respect and therefore to eat with respect. By using this method patients can see their desire to eat not as an occasion to feel deprived, but rather as one in which they are enhancing their mastery of the urge by choosing to protect their body.

Unfortunately, long-term outcome studies on the usefulness of hypnosis for weight control are lacking. There is evidence, however, from a randomized trial, that hypnosis increases weight loss treatment effectiveness (Barabasz & Spiegel, 1989). Clinical experience suggests that those within 20% of their ideal body weight may obtain some benefit from such restructuring techniques with self-hypnosis, when combined with a regimen of a balanced diet and exercise. Anderson (1985) reported that high hypnotizability is correlated with weight reduction.

## Conclusion

Hypnosis has been utilized to help with pain, anxiety, and to enhance control over somatic function for more than a century. It intensifies attention and extends brain control over body function, and brain response to sensory input. Techniques employing hypnosis are rapid, often effective, and rarely harmful. The oldest psychotherapy fits well with the newest biomedical treatments, and can be of benefit in coping with the growing problem of coping with chronic as well as acute medical illness.

## References

Andersen, M. S. (1985). Hypnotizability as a factor in the hypnotic treatment of obesity. *International Journal of Clinical and Experimental Hypnosis*, 33(2), 150–159.

Andreychuk, T., & Skriver, C. (1975). Hypnosis and biofeedback in the treatment of migraine headache. *The International Journal of Clinical and Experimental Hypnosis*, 23(3), 172–183.

Aronof, G. M., Aronoff, S., et al. (1975). Hypnotherapy in the treatment of bronchial asthma. *Annals of Allergy*, 42, 356–362.

Barabasz, A. F., Baer, L., et al. (1986). A three-year follow-up of hypnosis and restricted environmental stimulation therapy for smoking. *International Journal of Clinical and Experimental Hypnosis*, 34(3), 169–181.

Barabasz, M., & Spiegel, D. (1989). Hypnotizability and weight loss in obese subjects. *International Journal of Eating Disorders*, 8, 335–341.

Beecher, H. K. (1956). Relationship of significance of wound to pain experiences. *Journal of the American Medical Association*, 161, 1609–1613.

Berkowitz, B., Ross-Townsend, A., et al. (1979). Hypnotic treatment of smoking: the single-treatment method revisited. *American Journal of Psychiatry*, 136(1), 83–85.

Brose, W. G. & Spiegel, D. (1992). Neuropsychiatric aspects of pain management. In S. C. Yudofsky & R. E. Hales (Eds.), *The American Psychiatric Press Textbook of Neuropsychiatry* (pp. 245–275). Washington, D.C.: American Psychiatric Press, Inc.

Butler, L. D., Symons, B. K., et al. (2005). Hypnosis reduces distress and procedural time for children undergoing an invasive medical procedure. *Pediatrics*, 15(1), 77–85.

Calvert, E. L., Houghton, L. A., et al. (2002). Long-term improvement in functional dyspepsia using hypnotherapy. *Gastroenterology*, 123, 1778–1785.

Colgan, S. M., Faragher, E. B., et al. (1988). Controlled trial of hypnotherapy in relapse prevention of duodenal ulceration. *The Lancet*, 1(8598), 1299–1300.

DePascalis, V. (1999). Psychophysiological correlates of hypnosis and hypnotic susceptibility. *International Journal of Clinical and Experimental Hypnosis*, 47, 117–143.

Eisenberg, D. M., Davis, R. B., et al. (1998). Trends in alternative medicine use in the United States, 1990–1997: Results of a follow-up national survey. *Journal of the American Medical Association*, 280, 1569–1575.

Ellenberger, H. F. (1970). *Discovery of the Unconscious: The History and Evolution of Dynamic Psychiatry*. New York: Basic Books.

Esdaile, J. (1846). *Hypnosis in medicine and surgery*. New York: Julian Press.

Ewer, T. C., & Stewart, D. E. (1986). Improvement in bronchial hyper-responsiveness in patients with moderate asthma after treatment with a hypnotic technique: A randomised controlled trial. *British Medical Journal*, 293(6555), 1129–1132.

Ewin, D. M. (1992). Hypnotherapy for warts (verruca vulgaris): 41 consecutive cases with 33 cures. *American Journal of Clinical Hypnosis*, 35(1), 1–10.

Frank, R. G., Umlauf, R. L., et al. (1986). Hypnosis and behavioral treatment in a worksite smoking cessation program. *Addictive Behaviors*, 11(1), 59–62.

Frischholz, E. J., Tryon, W. W., et al. (1980). The relationship between the Hypnotic Induction Profile and the Stanford Hypnotic Susceptibility Scale, Form C: A replication. *American Journal of Clinical Hypnosis*, 22(4), 185–196.

Gardner, G., & Olness, K. (1981). *Hypnosis and Hypnotherapy with Children*. New York: Grune and Stratton.

Greenleaf, M., Fisher, S., et al. (1992). Hypnotizability and recovery from cardiac surgery. *American Journal of Clinical Hypnosis*, 35(2), 119–128.

Hyman, G. J., Stanley, R. O., et al. (1986). Treatment effectiveness of hypnosis and behaviour therapy in smoking cessation: A methodological refinement. *Addictive Behaviors*, 11(4), 355–365.

Kardiner, A., & Spiegel, H. (1947). *War Stress and Neurotic Illness*. New York: Paul Hoeber, Inc.

Katz, R., Kao, C.Y., et al. (1974). Acupuncture and hypnosis. *Advances in Neurology*, 4, 819–825.

Klein, K. B., & Spiegel, D. (1989). Modulation of gastric acid secretion by hypnosis. *Gastroenterology*, 96(6), 1383–1387.

Knox, V. J., & Shum, K. (1977). Reduction of cold-pressor pain with acupuncture analgesia in high- and low-hypnotic subjects. *Journal of Abnormal Psychology*, 86(6), 639–643.

Kohen, D. P., Olness, K., et al. (1984). The use of relaxation-mental imagery (self-hypnosis) in the management of 505 pediatric behavioral encounters. *Journal of Developmental and Behavioral Pediatrics*, 5(1), 21–25.

Kosslyn, S. M., Thompson, W. L., et al. (2000). Hypnotic visual illusion alters color processing in the brain. *American Journal of Psychiatry*, 157(8), 1279–1284.

Kuttner, L. (1988). Favorite stories: A hypnotic pain-reduction technique for children in acute pain. *American Journal of Clinical Hypnosis*, 30(4), 289–295.

Kuttner, L. (1989). Management of young children's acute pain and anxiety during invasive medical procedures. *Pediatrician*, 16(1–2), 39–44.

Kuttner, L. (1993). Managing pain in children. Changing treatment of headaches. *Canadian Family Practice*, 39, 563–568.

Lang, E. V., Benotsch, E. G., et al. (2000). Adjunctive non-pharmacological analgesia for invasive medical procedures: A randomised trial. *The Lancet*, 355, 1486–1490.

Lang, E. V. & Rosen, M. P. (2002). Cost analysis of adjunct hypnosis with sedation during outpatient interventional radiologic procedures. *Radiology*, 222(2), 375–382.

McGlashan, T. H., Evans, F. J., et al. (1969). The nature of hypnotic analgesia and placebo response to experimental pain. *Psychosomatic Medicine*, 31(3), 227–246.

Morrison, J. B. (1988). Chronic asthma and improvement with relaxation induced by hypnotherapy. *Journal of the Royal Society of Medicine*, 81(12), 701–704.

NIH Technology Assessment Panel (1996). Integration of behavioral and relaxation approaches into the treatment of chronic pain and insomnia. *Journal of the American Medical Association*, 276(4), 313–318.

Orne, M. T., Hilgard, E. R., et al. (1979). The relation between the Hypnotic Induction Profile and the Stanford Hypnotic Susceptibility Scales, Forms A and C. *International Journal of Clinical and Experimental Hypnosis*, 27, 85–102.

Rainville, P., Bushnell, M. C., et al. (2001). Representation of acute and persistent pain in the human CNS: Potential implications for chemical intolerance. *Annals of the New York Academy of Sciences*, 933, 130–141.

Rainville, P., Carrier, B., et al. (1999). Dissociation of sensory and affective dimensions of pain using hypnotic modulation. *Pain*, 82(2), 159–171.

Rainville, P., Duncan, G. H., et al. (1997). Pain affect encoded in human anterior cingulate but not somatosensory cortex. *Science*, 277(5328), 968–971.

Rainville, P., Hofbauer, R. K., et al. (2002). Hypnosis modulates activity in brain structures involved in the regulation of consciousness. *Journal of Cognitive Neuroscience*, 14(6), 887–901.

Schwartz, J. L. (1987). *Smoking Cessation Methods: United States and Canada 1978–85.* Bethesda, MD: Division of Cancer Prevention and Control, National Cancer Institute.

Spanos, N. P., Stenstrom, R. J., et al. (1988). Hypnosis, placebo, and suggestion in the treatment of warts. *Psychosomatic Medicine*, 50(3), 245–260.

Spanos, N. P., Williams, V., et al. (1990). Effects of hypnotic, placebo, and salicylic acid treatments on wart regression. *Psychosomatic Medicine*, 52(1), 109–114.

Spiegel, D., Bierre, P., et al. (1989). Hypnotic alteration of somatosensory perception. *American Journal of Psychiatry*, 146(6), 749–754.

Spiegel, D., Bloom, J. R., et al. (1981). Group support for patients with metastatic cancer. A randomized outcome study. *Archives of General Psychiatry*, 38(5), 527–533.

Spiegel, D., & Bloom, J. R. (1983). Pain in metastatic breast cancer. *Cancer*, 52(2), 341–345.

Spiegel, D., Frischholz, E. J., et al. (1993). Predictors of smoking abstinence following a single-session restructuring intervention with self-hypnosis. *American Journal of Psychiatry*, 150(7), 1090–1097.

Spiegel, H. (1970). Termination of smoking by a single treatment. *Archives of Environmental Health*, 20(6), 736–742.

Spiegel, H. & Spiegel, D. (1987). *Trance and Treatment: Clinical Uses of Hypnosis.* Washington, D.C.: American Psychiatric Press, Inc.

Spiegel, H. & Spiegel, D. (2004). *Trance and Treatment: Clinical Uses of Hypnosis.* Washington, D.C.: American Psychiatric Press, Inc.

Weinstein, E. J., & Au, P. K. (1991). Use of hypnosis before and during angioplasty. *American Journal of Clinical Hypnosis*, 34, 29–37.

Whorwell, P. J., Prior, A., et al. (1984). Controlled trial of hypnotherapy in the treatment of severe refractory irritable-bowel syndrome. *The Lancet*, 2(8414), 1232–1234.

Whorwell, P. J., Prior, A., et al. (1987). Hypnotherapy in severe irritable bowel syndrome: Further experience. *Gut*, 28, 423–425.

Williams, J. M., & Hall, D. W. (1988). Use of single session hypnosis for smoking cessation. *Addictive Behaviors*,13(2), 205–208.

Zeltzer, L., & LeBaron, S. (1982). Hypnosis and nonhypnotic techniques for reduction of pain and anxiety during painful procedures in children and adolescents with cancer. *Journal of Pediatrics*, 101(6), 1032–1035.

Zeltzer, L., LeBaron, S., et al. (1984). The effectiveness of behavioral intervention for reduction of nausea and vomiting in children and adolescents receiving chemotherapy. *Journal of Clinical Oncology*, 2(6), 683–690.

# Chapter 2

# The Biology of Hypnosis*

*Bruce H. Lipton*

In 1952, a young British physician made a mistake. It was a mistake that was to bring short-lived scientific glory to Dr. Albert Mason. Mason tried to treat a 15-year-old boy's warts using hypnosis. Mason and other doctors had previously successfully used hypnosis to get rid of warts, but this was an especially tough case. The boy's leathery skin looked more like an elephant's hide than a human's, except for his chest, which had normal skin.

Mason's first hypnosis session focused on one arm. When the boy was in a hypnotic trance, Mason told him that the skin on that arm would heal and turn into healthy, pink skin. When the boy came back a week later, Mason was gratified to see that the arm looked healthy. But when Mason brought the boy to the referring surgeon, who had unsuccessfully tried to help the boy with skin grafts, he learned that he had made a medical error. The surgeon's eyes were wide with astonishment when he saw the boy's arm. It was then that he told Mason that the boy was suffering, not from warts, but from a lethal genetic disease called congenital ichthyosis. By reversing the symptoms using "only" the power of the mind, Mason and the boy had accomplished what had until that time been considered impossible. Mason continued the hypnosis sessions, with the stunning result that most of the boy's skin came to look like the healthy, pink arm after the first hypnosis session. The boy, who had been mercilessly teased in school because of his grotesque-looking skin, went on to lead a normal life.

When Mason wrote about his startling treatment for ichthyosis in the *British Medical Journal* in 1952, his article created a sensation (Mason, 1952). Mason was touted in the media and became a magnet for patients suffering from the rare, lethal disease that no one before had ever cured. But hypnosis was in the end not a cure-all. Mason tried it on a number of other ichthyosis patients, but he was never able to replicate the results he had had with the young boy. Mason attributes his failure to his own *belief* about the treatment. When Mason treated

---

*This chapter is updated and adapted, by permission, from Chapter 5 of *Biology of Belief: Unleashing the Power of Consciousness, Matter and Miracles* (Lipton, 2005), Mountain of Love/Elite Books.

the new patients he couldn't replicate his cocky attitude as a young physician thinking he was treating a bad case of warts. After that first patient, Mason was fully aware that he was treating what everyone in the medical establishment knew to be a congenital, "incurable" disease. Mason tried to pretend that he was upbeat about the prognosis, but he told the Discovery Health Channel, "I was acting" (Discovery, 2003).

How is it possible that hypnosis can override genetic programming, as it did in the case above? And how could Mason's *belief* about that treatment affect its outcome? Exciting insights from the leading edge of biology provide some answers to the perennial questions concerning mind and body.

In the seventeenth century, René Descartes dismissed the idea that the mind influences the physical character of the body. Descartes' notion was that the physical body was made out of matter and the mind was made out of an unidentified, but clearly immaterial substance. Because he couldn't identify the nature of the mind, Descartes left behind an irresolvable philosophical conundrum: since only matter can affect matter, how can an immaterial mind be "connected" to a material body? The non-physical mind envisioned by Descartes was popularly defined as the "Ghost in the Machine" by Gilbert Ryle 50 years ago in his book *The Concept of Mind* (Ryle, 1949). Traditional biomedicine, whose science is based on a Newtonian matter-only universe, embraced Descartes' separation of mind and body. Medically speaking, it would be far easier to fix a mechanical body without having to deal with its meddling "ghost."

In contrast to the worldview of the matter-only Newtonian universe ascribed to by most life scientists, the reality of an energy-based quantum universe defined by physicists reconnects what Descartes took apart. Yes, the mind (energy) arises from the physical body, just as Descartes thought. However, our new understanding of quantum physics, the universe's mechanics, shows us how the physical body can be affected by the immaterial mind.

Biologists in the main have still not recognized the importance of quantum physics, but research suggests that sooner or later they will have to because the weight of scientific evidence is toppling the old materialist paradigm. An article by V. Pophristic and L. Goodman in the journal *Nature* in 2000 revealed that the laws of quantum physics, not Newtonian laws, control the life-generating movements of biologic molecules.

Reviewing this ground-breaking study for *Nature*, biophysicist F. Weinhold concluded: "When will chemistry textbooks begin to serve as aids, rather than barriers, to this enriched quantum-mechanic perspective on how molecular turnstiles work?" He further emphasized: "What are the forces that control the twisting and folding of molecules into complex shapes? Don't look for the answers in your organic chemistry textbook" (Weinhold, 2001). Yet organic chemistry provides the mechanistic foundation for biomedicine; and as Weinhold notes, that branch of science is so far out of date that its textbooks have yet to recognize quantum mechanics. Conventional medical researchers have no understanding of the molecular mechanisms that truly provide for life.

Hundreds upon hundreds of other scientific studies over the last 50 years have consistently revealed that "invisible forces" of the electromagnetic spectrum profoundly impact every facet of biological regulation. These energies include microwaves, radio frequencies, the visible light spectrum, extremely low frequencies, acoustic frequencies and even a newly recognized form of force known as scalar energy. Specific frequencies and patterns of electromagnetic radiation regulate DNA, RNA and protein syntheses, alter protein shape and function, and control gene regulation, cell division, cell differentiation, morphogenesis (the process by which cells assemble into organs and tissues), hormone secretion, nerve growth and function. Each one of these cellular activities is a fundamental behavior that contributes to the unfolding of life. Though these research studies have been published in some of the most respected mainstream biomedical journals, their revolutionary findings have not been incorporated into the medical school curriculum (Liboff, 2004; Goodman & Blank, 2002; Sivitz, 2000; Jin et al., 2000; Blackman et al., 1993; Rosen, 1992; Blank, 1992; Tsong, 1989; Yen-Patton et al., 1988).

An important study 40 years ago by Oxford University biophysicist C. W. F. McClare calculated and compared the efficiency of information transfer between energy signals and chemical signals in biological systems. His research, "Resonance in Bioenergetics" published in the *Annals of the New York Academy of Science*, revealed that energetic signaling mechanisms such as electromagnetic frequencies are a hundred times more efficient in relaying environmental information than physical signals such as hormones, neurotransmitters, growth factors and so on (McClare, 1974).

It is not surprising that energetic signals are so much more efficient. In physical molecules, the information that can be carried is directly linked to a molecule's available energy. However, the chemical coupling employed to transfer their information is accompanied by a massive loss of energy due to the heat generated in making and breaking chemical bonds. Because thermo-chemical coupling wastes most of the molecule's energy, the small amount of energy that remains limits the amount of information that can be carried as the signal.

We know that living organisms must receive and interpret environmental signals in order to stay alive. In fact, survival is directly related to the speed and efficiency of signal transfer. The speed of electromagnetic energy signals is 186,000 miles per second, while the speed of a diffusible chemical is considerably less than 1 centimeter per second. Energy signals are 100 times more efficient and infinitely faster than physical chemical signaling. What kind of signaling would a trillion-celled community prefer?

Thoughts, conceptualizations manifest through the mind's energy, directly influence how the physical brain controls the body's physiology. Thought "energy" can activate or inhibit the cell's function-producing proteins via the mechanics of constructive and destructive interference of interacting energy waves. We should examine the consequences of the energy we invest in our thoughts as closely as we examine the expenditures of energy we use to empower our physical bodies.

Despite the discoveries of quantum physics, the mind–body split in Western medicine still prevails. Scientists have been trained to dismiss cases like the boy above who used his mind to heal a genetically "predetermined" disease, as anomalies. In contrast, scientists should embrace the study of these anomalies. Buried in exceptional cases are the roots of a more powerful understanding of the nature of life – "more powerful" because the principles behind these exceptions trump established "truths." The fact is that harnessing the power of our minds can be *more* effective than the drugs we have been programmed to believe we need.

Before discussing the incredible power of our minds and how my research on cells provided insight into how the body's mind–body pathways work, I need to make it very clear that I do not believe that simply thinking positive thoughts necessarily leads to physical cures. You need more than just "positive thinking" to harness control of your body and your life. It *is* important for our health and well-being to shift the mind's energy toward positive, life-generating thoughts and eliminate ever-present, energy-draining and debilitating negative thoughts. But, and I mean that in the biggest sense of "BUT," the mere thinking of positive thoughts will not necessarily have any impact on our lives at all! In fact, sometimes people who "flunk" positive thinking become *more* debilitated because now they think their situation is hopeless – they believe they have exhausted all mind and body remedies.

What those positive-thinking dropouts haven't understood is that the seemingly "separate" subdivisions of the mind, the *conscious* and the *subconscious* are interdependent processing centers. The conscious mind is the creative one, the one that can conjure up "positive thoughts." In contrast, the subconscious mind is a repository of stimulus-response tapes derived from instincts and learned experiences. The subconscious mind is strictly habitual; it will play the same behavioral responses to life's signals over and over again, much to our chagrin.

The subconscious mind processes approx. 20,000,000 environmental stimuli per second vs. 40 environmental stimuli interpreted by the conscious mind in the same second (Nørretranders,1998). The subconscious mind, one of the most powerful information processors known, specifically observes both the surrounding world and the body's internal awareness, reads the environmental cues and immediately engages previously acquired (learned) behaviors – all without the help, supervision or even awareness of the conscious mind.

When it comes to sheer neurological processing abilities, the subconscious mind is millions of times more powerful than the conscious mind. If the desires of the conscious mind conflict with the programs in the subconscious mind, which "mind" do you think will win out? An individual can repeat the positive affirmation that she is lovable over and over or that his cancer tumor will shrink, but if, as a child, the person heard over and over that she or he was worthless and sickly, those messages programmed in the subconscious mind will undermine the best conscious efforts to change life. But for the moment, be aware that there is hope even for those who used positive thinking and failed miserably.

## Mind over Matter

Living organisms, from cells to human beings, survive through a complex integration of numerous physiologic systems, each providing a vital function, such as respiration, digestion, cardiovascular circulation, excretion, awareness and immune protection. To understand how each system "works," conventional biomedical sciences disassemble organisms to study their molecular components. Through this process of *reductionism*, science created the medical model, a belief that life is derived from a biochemical machine controlled by genes.

As a research scientist and former medical school professor, I actively supported and endorsed the fundamental belief that genes *control* life. The primacy of genes in the unfoldment of life is based upon one of science's most hallowed principles, the *Central Dogma*. The dogma, defined by Francis Crick, co-discoverer with James Watson of the genetic code, describes the flow of information in biological systems: DNA→RNA→Protein. Accordingly, genetic DNA blueprints, which codify our physical bodies, and consequently our lives, represent our *source*. Information encoded in the DNA is then translated into RNA molecules. The short-lived RNA versions of genes represent the actual molecular templates used in assembling proteins. Proteins are complex molecular building blocks that collectively form our bodies.

Based upon this dogma, the prevailing medical model emphasizes that the character and quality of human life is derived from the DNA programs comprising our genome. Our strengths, such as artistic or intellectual abilities, and our weaknesses, such as cardiovascular disease or depression, represent traits that are presumably preprogrammed in our genes. Thus we tend to perceive life's attributes and deficits, as well as our health and our frailties, as merely a reflection of heredity. This philosophy fosters the idea that both dysfunction and disease represent an inherent inability on the part the body to heal itself, and that remediation relies upon the administration of drugs – hence the name *medicine*.

Interestingly, the word *dogma* is defined as a belief that is based on religious reasoning rather than scientific fact. Astonishingly, the *Central Dogma*, the foundational pillar of conventional Science that declares *genes control life*, is actually a religious belief, one not based on science. Though the power of genes is still emphasized in current biology courses, textbooks and mass media, a radically new understanding is emerging at the frontiers of cell biology. New science clearly reveals that the Central Dogma is clearly unscientific! When mass consciousness fully integrates the exciting insights the "new" science offers on how life is controlled, the course of human civilization will be profoundly changed.

Interestingly, the first research revealing that genes did not *control* biology was published 100 years ago, long before the relevance of DNA was even understood. In those early days of cell research, many experimenters traced the fate of *enucleated* cells. Enucleation is the process of removing a cell's nucleus, the organelle that contains its genome. In many organisms, enucleated egg cells can divide and form a blastula, an embryological stage consisting of 40 or more cells, each of which possessed neither nuclei nor genes. Many enucleated, gene-less cells can survive for two or more months while maintaining strict regulation of their behavioral mechanisms. They maneuver through their world seeking food, digesting it and excreting wastes, breathing, avoiding toxins and socializing with other cells. If these cells possess no genes…then what *controls* their behavior?

While this awareness was in the domain of the experimental embryologist, it apparently never entered the realm of molecular genetics that myopically focused its attention on the genetic units of inheritance that Charles Darwin postulated controlled life. With the discovery of the universal genetic code by Watson and Crick, the putative power of DNA mesmerized the scientific world, blinding its inhabitants to alternative concepts of how life was controlled.

Until recently, it was thought that genes were *self-actualizing*…that genes could turn themselves on and off. Such behavior would be required in order for genes to *control* biology. Though the power of genes is still emphasized in current biology courses and textbooks, a radically new understanding of how life is controlled has emerged at the leading edge of cell science. It is now recognized that the environment, and more specifically, our *perception* (interpretation) of the environment, *directly* controls the activity of our genes. The environment controls gene activity through a process known as *epigenetic control*. Understanding the significance of epigenetic mechanisms requires that we review the nature of life and the hierarchy of its "control" mechanisms by starting from the bottom and working our way up.*

At the bottom level of life, the characteristic structures and behaviors of cells are derived from the assembly and function of their primary molecular building blocks, *proteins*. There are over 200 thousand different kinds of protein molecules used in making the cells and tissues of the human body. All proteins are the same in that they are all simple linear chains of linked amino acid molecules. The amino acid chain forms a flexible backbone that gives shape to the protein. There are 20 different amino acid subunits, each having a unique shape. Consequently, the specific sequence of different-shaped amino acids forming the backbone endows each protein with a unique structure.

Proteins are a special class of molecules for they express an unusual phenomenon – they can change their shape. The significance is that in changing shape, protein molecules move...in so doing, they express *behavior*. The collective activity of the cell's protein movements creates life. However, proteins only change shape in response to specific "activating" signals from the environment (in this case the environment means the whole *universe*).

When an environmental signal, which can be a physical/mechanical process, a chemical reaction or a specific resonant energy frequency, interacts with a protein it causes it to change its inherent molecular electrical charge. In response to alterations of the molecule's charge, the protein backbone flexes thereby causing the protein to change shape. Consequently, the behavior of a cell, which in turn represents the collective activity of its proteins, is a reflection of the signals the cell perceives from its environment. The behavior of the cell is a functional complement to the environment it finds itself in.

It is now recognized that genes are encased in a sleeve of *regulatory protein* molecules. The proteins comprising the gene's sleeve must change their shape and detach from the DNA in order for a gene to be exposed and activated. What causes a protein to change shape? Environmental signals. So what ultimately *controls* gene activity? Environmental signals. Cell behavior (protein movements) and gene activity are both regulated by the environmental signals *perceived* by the cell. Perception is the process by which a cell becomes aware of an environmental stimulus and then elicits a behavioral response. Perceptual mechanisms are housed in the structure of the cell's membrane, the interface

---

* The following description is an abridged version of the "new" biology, a further elaboration of which is freely downloadable from my website: www.brucelipton.com.

between environmental signals and the cell's behavior-producing cytoplasmic proteins.

The membrane provides a molecular mechanism that recognizes environmental stimuli and then engages appropriate, life-sustaining cellular responses. The cell membrane functions as the cell's "brain." Protein molecules built into the fabric of the membrane, called *integral membrane proteins* (IMPs), are the fundamental physical subunits of the cellular brain's "intelligence" mechanism. There are two principle classes of IMPs, receptor proteins and effector proteins. Receptors serve as protein antennas that respond to complementary environmental signals by changing their shape. The effectors are protein switches that engage cellular functions. In response to receiving a signal, an activated receptor protein changes its shape so that it complements an effector protein. The two proteins then couple, a process that activates the effector protein and enables it to control a specific cellular function. By definition, these membrane protein complexes represent "perception switches" that link reception of environmental stimuli to response-generating protein pathways.

Cells generally respond to a coterie of very basic "perceptions" of what's going on in their world. Such perceptions include whether things like potassium, calcium, oxygen, glucose, histamine, estrogen, toxins, light or any number of other stimuli are present in their immediate environment. The simultaneous interactions of tens of thousands of reflexive perception switches in the membrane, each directly reading an individual environmental signal, collectively create the complex behavior of a living cell.

## *The Hierarchy of Control*

For the first three billion years of life on this planet, the biosphere consisted of free-living single cells such as bacteria, algae and protozoans. While we have traditionally considered such life forms as solitary individuals, we are now aware that signal molecules used by individual cells to regulate their own physiologic functions also influence the behavior of other organisms. Signals released into the environment allow for a coordination of behavior among a dispersed population of unicellular organisms. Secreting signal molecules into the environment enhanced the survival of single cells by providing them with the opportunity to integrate their behaviors and live as a primitive "community."

The single-celled slime mold amoebas provide an example of how signaling molecules lead to community. These amoebas live a solitary existence in the soil foraging for food. When available food in the environment is consumed, the cells synthesize an excess amount of a metabolic byproduct called cyclic-AMP (cAMP), much of which is released into the environment. The concentration of the released cAMP builds in the environment as other amoeba face starvation. As the concentration of extracellular cAMP signals increases, the molecules bind to cAMP-receptors on the cell membranes of other slime mold amoeba. Cyclic-AMP binding causes the amoebas to activate a swarming behavior wherein they congregate and form a large multicellular "slug." The slug community is the reproductive stage of slime mold. During the "famine" period, the community of aging cells shares their DNA and creates the next generation of offspring. The new amoeba hibernate as inactive spores. When more food is available, the food molecules act as an environmental signal to break the hibernation, releasing a new population of single cells to start the cycle over again.

The point is that single-celled organisms actually live in community when they share their "awareness" and coordinate their behaviors by releasing "signal" molecules into the environment. Cyclic-AMP was one of evolution's earliest forms of secreted regulatory signals that control cell behavior. The fundamental human signal molecules (e.g., hormones, neuropeptides, cytokines, growth factors) that regulate our own cellular communities were once thought to have arisen with the appearance of complex multicellular life forms. However, recent research now reveals that primitive single-celled organisms were already using these "human" signal molecules in the earliest stages of evolution.

Through evolution, cells maximized the number of IMP "awareness" proteins their membranes could hold. To acquire more awareness, and therefore increase their probability of surviving, cells started to assemble, first into simple colonies and later into highly organized cellular communities. The physiologic functions of multicellular organisms are parceled out to specialized communities of cells forming the body's tissues and organs. In communal organizations, the specialized cells of the organism's nervous and immune systems carry out the cell membrane's intelligence processing function.

It was only 700 million years ago, recent within the context of life on this planet, when single cells found it advantageous to join together in tightly knit multicellular communities, organizations we recognize as animals and plants. The same coordinating signal molecules used by free-living cells were used in these newly evolved closed communities. By tightly regulating the release and distribution of these function-controlling signal molecules, the community of cells would be able to coordinate their functions and act as a single life form.

In more primitive multicellular organisms, those without specialized nervous systems, the flow of these signal molecules among the cells of the community provided an elementary "mind," represented by the coordinating information shared by every cell. In such organisms, each cell directly reads environmental cues and personally adjusts its own behavior.

However, when cells came together in community, a new politic had to be established. In community, each cell cannot act as an independent agent that does whatever it wants. The term "community" implies that all of its members commit to a common plan of action. Within multicellular animals, individual cells may "see" the local environment outside of their own "skin," but they may have no awareness of what is going on in more distant environments, especially those outside of the whole organism itself. Can a liver cell buried in your viscera, responding to its local environmental signals, make an informed response regarding the consequence of a mugger that jumps into your environment? The complex behavior controls needed to ensure a multicellular organization's survival are incorporated within its centralized information-processing system.

As more complex animals evolved, specialized cells took over the job of monitoring and organizing the flow of the behavior regulating signal molecules. These cells provided a distributed nerve network and central information processor, a brain. The brain's function is to coordinate the dialogue of signal molecules within the community. Consequently, in a community of cells, each cell must defer control to the informed decisions of its awareness authority, the *brain*. The brain *controls* the behavior of the body's cells. This is a very important point to consider as we continually blame the cells of our organs and tissues for the health issues we experience in our lives.

In higher, more aware life forms, the brain developed a specialization that enabled the whole community to tune into the status of its regulatory signals. The evolution of the limbic system provided a unique mechanism that converted the chemical communication signals into sensations that could be experienced by all of the cells in the community. Our conscious mind experiences these signals as *emotions*. The mind not only "reads" the flow of the cellular coordinating signals, it can also generate emotions, which are manifest through the controlled release of the same regulatory signals by the nervous system.

In *Molecules of Emotion* (1997), Candace Pert revealed how her study of information-processing receptors on nerve cell membranes led her to discover that the same "neural" receptors were present on most, if not all, of the body's cells. Her elegant experiments established that the "mind" was not focused in the head, but was distributed via signal molecules to the whole body. As important, her work emphasized that emotions were not only derived through a feedback of the body's environmental information. Through self-consciousness, the mind can use the brain to *generate* "molecules of emotion" and override the system. While proper use of consciousness can bring health to an ailing body, inappropriate unconscious control of emotions can easily make a healthy body dysfunctional.

The limbic system offered a major evolutionary advance through its ability to sense and coordinate the flow of behavior-regulating signals within the cellular community. As this internal signal system evolved, the greater efficiency it offered the body enabled the brain to physically increase in size. The brains of higher multicellular organisms gained increasingly more cells that were dedicated to responding to an ever-wider variety of *external* environmental signals. While individual cells can respond to simple sensory perceptions such as red, round, aromatic, and sweet, the extra brainpower available in multicellular animals enables them to combine those simple sensations into a higher level of complexity and perceive "apple."

Fundamental reflex behaviors acquired through evolution are passed on to offspring in the form of genetic-based instincts. The evolution of larger brains, with their increased neural cell population, offered organisms the opportunity not only to rely on instinctual behavior, but also to learn from their life experiences. The learning of novel reflex behaviors is essentially a product of *conditioning*. For example, consider the classic example of Pavlov training his dogs to salivate at the ring of a bell. He first trained them by ringing a bell and coupling that stimulus with a food reward. After a while, he would ring the bell but not offer the food. By that time, the dogs were so programmed to expect the food that when the bell rang, they reflexively started to salivate even though no food was present. This is clearly an "unconscious," learned reflex behavior.

Reflex behaviors may be as simple as the spontaneous kick of the leg when a mallet taps the knee, or as complex as driving a car at 65 miles per hour on a crowded interstate highway while your conscious mind is fully engaged in conversation with a passenger. Though conditioned behavioral responses may be inordinately complex, they are "no-brainers." Through conditioning, neural pathways between eliciting stimuli and behavioral responses become hardwired to ensure a repetitive pattern. Hardwired pathways are "habits." In lower animals, the entire brain is designed to engage in purely habitual responses to stimuli. Pavlov's dogs salivate by reflex...not by deliberate intention. The actions of the subconscious mind are reflexive in nature and are not governed by reason or thinking. Physically, the "subconscious mind" is associated with the function of the whole brain in animals that have not evolved self-consciousness.

Humans and a number of other higher mammals have evolved a specialized region of the brain associated with thinking, planning and decision-making called the prefrontal cortex. This portion of the forebrain is apparently the seat of the "self-conscious" mind processing. The self-conscious mind is self-reflective; it is a newly evolved "sense organ" that senses our emotions and observes our own behaviors. The self-conscious mind also has access to most of the data stored in the subconscious' long-term memory bank. This is an extremely important feature allowing our history of life to be considered as we consciously plan our futures.

Endowed with the ability to be self-reflective, the self-conscious mind is extremely powerful. It can observe any programmed behavior we are engaged in, evaluate the behavior and consciously decide to change the program. We can actively *choose* how to respond to most environmental signals and whether or not we even want to respond at all. The conscious mind's capacity to override the subconscious mind's preprogrammed behaviors is the foundation of free will.

However, our special gift comes with a special pitfall. While almost all organisms have to actually experience the stimuli of life firsthand, the human brain's ability to "learn" perceptions is so advanced that we can actually acquire perceptions indirectly from teachers. Once we accept the perceptions of others as "truths," *their* perceptions become hardwired into our own brains, becoming *our* "truths."

Here's where the problem arises: what if the perceptions of our teachers are inaccurate? In such cases, our brains are then downloaded with *misperceptions*. The subconscious mind is strictly a stimulus-response playback device; there is no "ghost" in that part of the "machine" to ponder the long-term consequences of the programs we engage. The subconscious works only in the "now." Consequently, programmed misperceptions in our subconscious mind are not "monitored" and will habitually engage us in inappropriate and limiting behaviors.

If I included as a bonus in this chapter a slithering snake that pops out of this page right now, most of you would run from the room or throw the book out of the house. Whoever "introduced" you to your first snake may have behaved in such a shocked way as to give your impressionable mind an apparently important life lesson: See snake...snake baaad! The subconscious memory system is very partial to rapidly downloading and emphasizing perceptions regarding things in your environment that are threatening to life and limb. If you were taught that snakes are dangerous, any time a snake comes into your proximity, you will reflexively (unconsciously) engage in a protective response.

But what if a herpetologist were reading this book and a snake popped out? No doubt herpetologists would not only be intrigued by the snake, they would be *thrilled* with the bonus included in the book. They would then hold it and watch its behaviors with delight. They would think that *your* programmed response was an irrational one, because not all snakes are dangerous. Further they would be saddened by the fact that so many people are deprived of the pleasure of studying such interesting creatures. Same snake, same stimulus, yet greatly different responses.

Our responses to environmental stimuli are indeed controlled by perceptions, but not all of our learned perceptions are accurate. Not all snakes are dangerous! Yes, perception "controls" biology, but as we've seen, these perceptions can be true or false. Therefore, we would be more accurate to refer to these controlling perceptions as *beliefs*.

## Beliefs control biology!

Ponder the significance of this information. We have the capacity to consciously evaluate our responses to environmental stimuli and change old responses any time we desire…once we deal with the powerful subconscious mind. We are not stuck with our genes or our self-defeating behaviors!

My insights into how beliefs control biology are grounded in my studies of cloned endothelial cells, the cells that line the blood vessels. The endothelial cells I grew in culture monitor their world closely and change their behavior based on information they pick up from the environment. When I provided nutrients, the cells would gravitate toward those nutrients with the cellular equivalent of open arms. When I created a toxic environment, the cultured cells would retreat from the stimulus in an effort to wall themselves off from the noxious agents. My research focused on the membrane perception switches that controlled the shift from one behavior to the other.

The primary switch I was studying has a protein receptor that responds to histamine, a molecule that the body uses in a way that is equivalent to a local emergency alarm. I found that there are two varieties of switches, H1 and H2, which respond to the same histamine signal. When activated, switches with H1 histamine receptors evoke a *protection response*, the type of behavior revealed by cells in toxin-containing culture dishes. Switches containing H2 histamine receptors evoke a *growth response* to histamine, similar to the behavior of cells cultured in the presence of nutrients.

I subsequently learned that the body's system-wide emergency response signal, adrenaline, also has switches sporting two different adrenaline-sensing receptors, called *alpha* and *beta*. The adrenaline receptors provoked the exact same cell behaviors as those elicited by histamine. When the adrenal *alpha*-receptor is part of an IMP switch, it provokes a protection response when adrenaline is perceived. When the *beta*-receptor is part of the switch, the same adrenaline signal activates a growth response (Lipton et al., 1992).

All that was interesting, but the most exciting finding was when I simultaneously introduced both histamine and adrenaline into my tissue cultures. I found that adrenaline signals, released by the central nervous system, override the influence of histamine signals that are produced locally. This is where the politics of the community described earlier comes into play. Suppose you're working in a bank. The branch manager gives you an order. The CEO walks in and gives you the opposite order. Which order would you follow? If you want to keep your job, you'll snap to the CEO's order. There is a similar priority built into our biology, which requires cells to follow instructions from the head honcho nervous system, even if those signals are in conflict with local stimuli.

I was excited by these experiments because I believed that they revealed on the single-cell level a truth for multicellular organisms – that the mind (i.e., acting via the central nervous system's adrenaline) overrides the body (acting via the local histamine signal). I wanted to spell out the implications of my experiments in my research paper, but my colleagues almost died from apoplexy at the notion of injecting the body–mind connection into a paper about cell biology. So, I put in a cryptic comment about understanding the significance of the study, but I couldn't say what the significance was. My colleagues did not want me to include these implications of my research because the mind is not an acceptable biological concept. Bioscientists are conventional Newtonians – if it isn't matter…it doesn't matter. The "mind" is a non-localized energy and therefore is not relevant to materialistic biology. Unfortunately, that perception is a "belief" that has been proven to be patently incorrect in a quantum mechanical universe!

## Placebos: The Belief Effect

Every medical student learns, at least in passing, that the mind can affect the body. They learn that some people get better when they *believe* (falsely) they are getting medicine. When patients get better by ingesting a sugar pill, medicine defines it as the *placebo effect*. I call it the *belief effect* to stress that our perceptions, whether they are accurate or inaccurate, equally impact our behavior and our bodies.

I celebrate the *belief effect*, which is an amazing testament to the healing ability of the body/mind. However, the "all in their minds" placebo effect has been linked by traditional medicine to, at worst, quacks or, at best, weak, suggestible patients. The placebo effect is quickly glossed over in medical schools so that students can get to the *real* tools of modern medicine like drugs and surgery.

This is a mistake. The placebo effect should be a major topic of study in medical school. Medical education should train doctors to recognize the power of our internal resources. Doctors should not dismiss the power of the mind as something inferior to the power of chemicals and the scalpel. They should let go of their conviction that the body and its parts are essentially stupid and that we need outside intervention to maintain our health

The placebo effect should be the subject of major funded research efforts. If medical researchers could figure out how to leverage the placebo effect, they would hand doctors an efficient, energy-based, side effect-free tool to treat dysfunction. Energy healers say they already have such tools, but as a scientist I believe the more we know about the science of the placebo, the better we'll be able to use it in clinical settings.

The reason the mind has so summarily been dismissed in medicine is the result, not only of dogmatic thinking, but also of financial considerations. If the power of your mind can heal your sick body, why would you go to the doctor and *more* important, why would you need to buy drugs? In fact, I was recently disturbed to learn that drug companies are studying patients who respond to sugar pills with the goal of *eliminating* them from early clinical trials. Pharmaceutical manufacturers are always upset by the fact that in most of their clinical trials the placebos, the "fake" drugs, prove to be as effective as their engineered chemical cocktails (Greenberg, 2003). Though the drug companies insist they're not trying to make it easier for ineffective drugs to get approved, it is clear that the effectiveness of placebo pills are a threat to the pharmaceutical industry. The message from the drug companies is clear: if you can't beat placebo pills fairly, simply remove the competition.

The fact that most doctors are not trained to consider the impact of the placebo effect is ironic because some historians make a strong case that the history of medicine is largely the history of the placebo effect. For most of medical history, doctors did not have effective methods to fight disease. Some of the more notorious treatments once prescribed by mainstream medicine include bloodletting, treating wounds with arsenic and the proverbial cure-all, rattlesnake oil. No doubt some patients, the conservatively estimated one-third of the population who are particularly susceptible to the healing power of the placebo effect, got better with those treatments. In today's world, when doctors wearing white coats deliver a treatment decisively, patients may *believe* the treatment works – and so it does, whether it is a real drug or just a sugar pill.

Though the question of *how* placebos work has generally been ignored by medicine, recently some mainstream medical researchers have been turning their attention to it. The results of those studies suggest that it is not only off the wall, nineteenth-century treatments that can foster a placebo effect but also modern medicine's sophisticated technology, including the most "concrete" of medical tools, surgery.

A Baylor School of Medicine study, published in 2002 in the *New England Journal of Medicine* evaluated surgery for patients with severe, debilitating knee pain (Moseley et al., 2002). The lead author of the study, Dr. Bruce Moseley, "knew" that knee surgery helped his patients: "All good surgeons know there is no placebo effect in surgery." But Moseley was trying to figure out which part of the surgery was giving his patients relief. The patients in the study were divided into three groups. Moseley shaved the damaged cartilage in the knee of one group. For another group, he flushed out the knee joint, removing material thought to be causing the inflammatory effect. Both of these options constitute standard treatment for arthritic knees. The third group got "fake" surgery. The patient was sedated, Moseley made three standard incisions and then talked and acted just as he would have during a real surgery – he even splashed salt water to simulate the sound of the knee-washing procedure. After 40 minutes, Moseley sewed up the incisions as if he had done the surgery. All three groups were prescribed the same postoperative care, which included an exercise program.

The results were shocking. Yes, the groups who received surgery, as expected, improved. But the placebo group improved just as much as the other two groups. Despite the fact that there are 650,000 surgeries yearly for arthritic knees, at a cost of about $5,000 each, the results were clear to Moseley: "My skill as a surgeon had no benefit on these patients. The entire benefit of surgery for osteo-arthritis of the knee was the placebo effect." Television news programs graphically illustrated the stunning results. Footage showed members of the placebo group walking and playing basketball, in short doing things they reported they could not do before their "surgery." The placebo patients didn't find out for two years that they had gotten fake surgery. One member of the placebo group, Tim Perez, who had to walk with a cane before the surgery, is now able to play basketball with his grandchildren. He summed up the theme of this book when he told the Discovery Health Channel: "In this world anything is possible when you put your mind to it. I know that your mind can work miracles."

Studies have shown the placebo effect to be powerful in treating other diseases, including asthma and Parkinson's. In the treatment of depression, placebos are stars; in fact, psychiatrist Walter Brown of the Brown University School of Medicine has proposed placebo pills as the first treatment for patients with mild or moderate depression (Brown, 1998). Patients would be told that they'd be receiving a remedy with no active ingredient, but that it shouldn't dampen the pills' effectiveness. Studies suggest that even when people know they're not getting a drug, the placebo pills still work.

One indication of the power of the placebo came from a recent report from the United States Department of Health and Human Services. The report found that half of severely depressed patients taking drugs improve versus 32 percent taking a placebo (Horgan, 1999). Even this impressive showing may under-estimate the power of the placebo effect because many study participants figure out they're taking the real drug based on side-effects that are not experienced by those taking the placebo. Once those patients realize they're taking the drug – once they start *believing* that they're getting the *real* pill – they are even more susceptible to the placebo effect.

Given the power of the placebo, it is no wonder that the $8.2 billion antidepressant industry is under attack by critics who charge that drug companies are hyping the effectiveness of their pills. In a 2002 article in the American Psychological Association's *Prevention & Treatment*, "The Emperor's New Drugs," University of Connecticut psychology professor Irving Kirsch found that 80 percent of the effect of antidepressants, as measured in clinical trials, could be attributed to the placebo effect (Kirsch et al., 2002). Kirsch had to invoke the Freedom of Information Act in 2001 to acquire information on the clinical trials of the top antidepressants: the data were not forthcoming from the Food and Drug Administration. The data show that in more than half of the clinical trials for the six leading antidepressants, the drugs did not outperform placebo, sugar pills. And Kirsch noted in a Discovery Health Channel interview: "The difference between the response of the drugs and the response of placebo was less than two points on average on this clinical scale that goes from 50 to 60 points. That's a very small difference. That difference clinically is meaningless."

Another interesting fact about the effectiveness of antidepressants is that they have performed better and better in clinical trials over the years, suggesting that their placebo effects are in part due to savvy marketing. The more the miracle of antidepressants was touted in the media and in advertisements, the more effective they became. Beliefs are contagious. We now live in a culture where people *believe* that antidepressants work, and so they do.

A California interior designer, Janis Schonfeld, who took part in a clinical trial to test the efficacy of Effexor in 1997, was just as "stunned" as Perez when she found out that she had been on a placebo. Not only had the pills relieved her of the depression that had plagued her for 30 years, the brain scans she received throughout the study found that the activity of her prefrontal cortex was greatly enhanced (Leuchter et al., 2002). Her improvements were not "all in her head." When the mind changes it absolutely affects your biology. Schonfeld also experienced nausea, a common Effexor side effect. She is typical of patients who improve with placebo treatment and then find out they were not on the real drug – she was convinced the doctors had made a mistake in the labeling because she "knew" she was on the drug. She insisted that the researchers double-check their records to make absolutely sure she wasn't on the drug.

While many in the medical profession are aware of the placebo effect, few have considered its implications for self-healing. If positive thinking can pull you out of depression and heal a damaged knee, consider what negative thinking can do in your life. When the mind, through positive suggestion improves health, it is referred to as the placebo effect. Conversely, when the same mind is engaged in negative suggestions that can damage health, the negative effects are referred to as the *nocebo* effect.

In medicine, the nocebo effect can be as powerful as the placebo effect, a fact everyone should keep in mind every time they step into a doctor's office. By their words and their demeanor, physicians can convey hope-deflating messages to their patients, messages that are, I believe, completely unwarranted. Albert Mason, for example, thinks his inability to project optimism to his patients hampered his efforts with his ichthyosis patients. Another example is the potential power of the statement: "You have six months to live." If one chooses to believe the doctor's message, one is not likely to have much more time on this planet.

I have cited the Discovery Health Channel's 2003 program "Placebo: Mind Over Medicine" because it is a good compendium of some of medicine's most interesting cases. One of its more poignant segments featured a Nashville physician, Clifton Meador, who has been reflecting on the potential power of the nocebo effect for 30 years. In 1974 Meador had a patient, Sam Londe, a retired shoe salesman suffering from cancer of the esophagus, a condition that was at the time considered 100 percent fatal. Londe was treated for that cancer but everyone in the medical community "knew" that his esophageal cancer would recur. So, it was no surprise when Londe died a few weeks after his diagnosis.

The surprise came after Londe's death when an autopsy found very little cancer in his body, certainly not enough to kill him. There were a couple of spots in the liver and one in the lung, but there was no trace of the esophageal cancer that everyone thought had killed him. Meador told the Discovery Health Channel: "He died with cancer, but not from cancer." What did Londe die of if not esophageal cancer? Had he died because he *believed* he was going to die? The case still haunts Meador three decades after Londe's death: "I thought he had cancer. He thought he had cancer. Everybody around him thought he had cancer...did I remove hope in some way?" Troublesome nocebo cases suggest that physicians, parents and teachers can remove hope by programming us to believe we are powerless.

Our positive and negative beliefs not only impact our health, but also every aspect of our life. Henry Ford was right about the efficiency of assembly lines and he was right about the power of the mind: "If you believe you can or if you believe you can't...you're right." Beliefs act like filters on a camera, changing how we see the world. And our biology adapts to those beliefs. When we truly recognize that our beliefs are that powerful, we hold the key to freedom. While we cannot readily change the codes of our genetic blueprints, we can change our minds.

The subconscious mind is a programmable autopilot that can navigate the "vehicle" without the observation or awareness of the pilot – the conscious mind. When the subconscious autopilot is controlling behavior, consciousness is free to dream into the future or review the past. The dual-mind system's effectiveness is defined by the quality of the programs carried in the subconscious mind. Essentially, the person who taught us to "drive" molds our driving skills. For example, if we are taught to drive with one foot on the gas and the other on the brake, no matter how many vehicles we own, each will inevitably express premature brake and engine failure. Similarly, if our subconscious mind is programmed with inappropriate behavioral responses to life's experiences, then our sub-optimum "driving skills" will contribute to a life of crash-and-burn experiences. Cardiovascular disease, for example, one of the leading causes of death, is directly attributable to behavioral programs that mismanage the body's response to stress.

Are we good drivers or bad drivers? The answer is difficult for in our conscious creative mind we may consider ourselves to be good drivers, however, self-sabotaging or limiting behavioral programs in our subconscious secretly undermine our efforts. We are generally consciously unaware of our fundamental perceptions or beliefs about life. The reason is that the prenatal and neonatal brain is predominately operating in *delta* and *theta* EEG frequencies through the first six years of our lives. This low level of brain activity is associated with the hypnogogic state. While in this hypnotic trance, children do not have to be actively coached by their parents for they obtain their behavioral programs simply by observing their parents, siblings, peers and teachers. The question then concerns whether one's early developmental experiences provided good models of behavior to use in the unfolding of life.

During the first six years of life, a child unconsciously acquires the behavioral repertoire needed to become a functional member of society. In addition, a child's subconscious mind also downloads beliefs relating to "self." When a parent tells a young child it is stupid, undeserving or any other negative trait, this is hypnotically downloaded as a "fact" into the youngster's subconscious mind. These acquired beliefs constitute the "central voice" that controls the fate of the body's cellular community. While the conscious mind may hold one's self in high regard, the more powerful unconscious mind may simultaneously engage in self-destructive behavior.

The insidious part of the autopilot mechanism is that subconscious behaviors are programmed to engage without the control of, or observation by, the conscious self. Since most of our behaviors are under the control of the subconscious mind, we rarely observe them or much less know that they are even engaged. While the conscious mind perceives that one is a good driver, the unconscious mind that has its hands on the wheel most of the time, may be driving down the road to ruin.

The beliefs wired into the subconscious mind act as "filters" through which our perceptions of the world are interpreted. To demonstrate the power of these belief "filters'" in my lectures, I provide two sets of plastic filters, one red and one green. I have the audience pick one color and then look at a blank screen through the filter. I then tell them to yell out whether the image I project next is one that generates love or generates fear. Those in the audience who don the red "belief" filters see an inviting picture of a cottage labeled "House of Love," flowers, a sunny sky and the message "I live in Love." Those wearing the green filters see a threatening dark sky, bats, snakes, a ghost hovering outside a dark, gloomy house and the words "I live in fear." I always get enjoyment out of seeing how the audience responds to the confusion when half yell out "I live in love," and the other half, in equal certainty, yells out "I live in fear" in response to the same image.

Then I ask the audience to change to the opposite colored filters. My point is that you can choose what to see. We can filter our lives with rose-colored beliefs that will help our bodies grow or we can use a dark filter that turns everything black and makes our body/mind more susceptible to disease. We can live a life of fear or live a life of love. We have the choice! But I can tell you that if we choose to see a world full of love, our bodies will respond by growing in health. If we choose to believe that we live in a dark world full of fear, our bodies' health will be compromised as we physiologically close ourselves down in a protection response.

As conventional science comes to fully accept the relationship between thoughts and biological expression, primary health care will likely focus on identifying and reprogramming limiting beliefs programmed into our subconscious mind. It is the recognition of this singular point that will ultimately catapult hypnotherapy to its rightful role as a preeminent modality in the healing arsenal. Hypnotherapists actively intervene in rewriting the database of the client's learned beliefs. By facilitating change in the patient's *perception* of his or her environment, the therapist directly participates in the production of new belief "filters" through which the patient views life. By facilitating the programming of a healthy, supportive environment, hypnotherapy can help individuals select physiological programs that support their growth and cancel self-destructive pathological behaviors (physiology) elicited by negative developmental programming.

In conclusion, we are poised on the threshold of radical revision of basic bio-medical thought. Rather than perceiving our health and behavior as a consequence of our genetic heritage, we will soon recognize that we are masters of our fate. All that is necessary is that we own the reality that we are the physical expression of our beliefs. Inevitably, hypnotherapists, by their ability to modify these influential beliefs, will be acknowledged as one of the primary caregivers in human civilization.

Learning how to harness our minds to promote growth is the secret of life, which is why I refer to the new science as the *Biology of Belief.* Of course the secret of life is not a secret at all. Teachers like Buddha and Jesus have been telling us the same story for millennia. Now science is pointing in the same direction. It is not our genes but our beliefs that control our lives…Oh ye of little belief!

# References

Blackman, C. F., Benane, S. G., et al. (1993). Evidence for direct effect of magnetic fields on neurite outgrowth. *Federation of American Societies for Experimental Biology, 7,* 801–806.

Blank, M. (1992). Na,K-ATPase function in alternating electric fields. *75th Annual Meeting of the Federation of American Societies for Experimental Biology*, April 23, Atlanta, Georgia.

Brown, W. A. (1998). The Placebo Effect: Should doctors be prescribing sugar pills? *Scientific American, 278*(1), 90–95.

DiRita, V. J. (2000). Genomics happens. *Science, 289,* 1488–1489.

Discovery (2003). Placebo: Mind over medicine? Medical Mysteries. Silver Spring, MD: Discovery Health Channel.

Goodman, R., & Blank, M. (2002). Insights into electromagnetic interaction mechanisms. *Journal of Cellular Physiology*, 192, 16–22.

Greenberg, G. (2003). Is it Prozac? Or placebo? *Mother Jones,* 76–81.

Horgan, J. (1999). *The Undiscovered Mind: How the Human Brain Defies Replication, Medication, and Explanation.* New York: The Free Press.

Jin, M., Blank, M., et al. (2000). ERK1/2 Phosphorylation, induced by electromagnetic fields, diminishes during neoplastic transformation. *Journal of Cell Biology,* 78, 371–379.

Kirsch, I., Moore, T. J., et al. (2002). The emperor's new drugs: An analysis of antidepressant medication data submitted to the U.S. Food and Drug Administration. *Prevention & Treatment (American Psychological Association),* 5, Article 23.

Leuchter, A. F., Cook, I. A., et al. (2002). Changes in brain function of depressed subjects during treatment with placebo. *American Journal of Psychiatry,* 159(1), 122–129.

Liboff, A. R. (2004). Toward an electromagnetic paradigm for biology and medicine. *Journal of Alternative and Complementary Medicine,* 10(1), 41–47.

Lipton, B. H., Bensch, K. G., et al. (1992). Histamine-modulated transdifferentiation of dermal microvascular endothelial cells. *Experimental Cell Research, 199,* 279–291.

McClare, C. W. F. (1974). Resonance in bioenergetics. *Annals of the New York Academy of Sciences, 227,* 74–97.

Mason, A. A. (1952). A case of congenital ichthyosiform erythrodermia of brocq treated by hypnosis. *British Medical Journal, 30,* 442–443.

Moseley, J. B., O'Malley, K., et al. (2002). A controlled trial of arthroscopic surgery for osteoarthritis of the knee. *New England Journal of Medicine, 347*(2), 81–88.

Nørretranders, T. (1998). *The User Illusion: Cutting Consciousness Down to Size.* New York: Penguin Books.

Pert, Candace (1997). *Molecules of Emotion: The Science Behind Mind–Body Medicine.* New York: Scribner.

Pophristic, V., & Goodman, L. (2001). Hyperconjugation not steric repulsion leads to the staggered structure of ethane. *Nature, 411,* 565–568.

Rosen, A. D. (1992). Magnetic field influence on acetylcholine release at the neuromuscular junction. *American Journal of Physiology-Cell Physiology, 262,* C1418–C1422.

Ryle, G. (1949). *The Concept of Mind.* Chicago: University of Chicago Press.

Sivitz, L. (2000). Cells proliferate in magnetic fields. *Science News, 158,* 195.

Tsong, T. Y. (1989). Deciphering the language of cells. *Trends in Biochemical Sciences, 14,* 89–92.

Weinhold, F. (2001). A new twist on molecular shape. *Nature, 411,* 539–541.

Yen-Patton, G. P. A., Patton, W.F., et al. (1988). Endothelial cell response to pulsed electromagnetic fields: Stimulation of growth rate and angiogenesis in vitro. *Journal of Cellular Physiology, 134,* 37–46.

## Chapter 3

# *Hypnotic Induction Profile*

*David Spiegel and George Fraser*

The Hypnotic Induction Profile (HIP) was developed by Drs. Herbert and David Spiegel. They point out that the ability to enter a hypnotic trance varies in the population basically as a bell-shaped distribution curve. A smaller number are low responders, the majority are fairly good responders, and at the other end of this curve is again a smaller number who are very high hypnotic responders.

There are various tests devised to measure this innate hypnotic capacity, one of which is the HIP. The benefit of the HIP is that it is brief (about six minutes) and can easily be done in the therapist's office. The HIP is a standardized procedure that provides a reliable measure of a subject's ability to use this capacity in a clinical setting. The scores also provide a basis for clinicians to convey that client's hypnotic capacity to other clinicians who may be working with the client concurrently or at a later date. Measuring hypnotic capacity can provide valuable information in assessing how much trance capacity may be influencing the clinical presentation (generally greater in high hypnotic responders, and less likely in low or moderate responders) even before formal hypnosis is utilized.

Many therapists do not perform measurements or scales for assessing hypnotic capacity. Others feel that it is useful and many around the world have chosen the HIP as a user-friendly way of measuring trance capacity and introducing hypnosis as a therapeutic modality. As well, such measurements may provide an objective measurement when hypnosis is used in research. The following material on HIP will offer useful details regarding this popular clinical measurement.

## The Hypnotic Induction Profile

The Hypnotic Induction Profile (HIP) is a measurement of hypnotizability in which a systematized sequence of instructions, responses, and observations are recoded with a uniform momentum in a standardized way, as the subject shifts into trance to the extent of his or her ability, maintains it, and then exits in a prescribed manner (Spiegel & Spiegel, 2004).

Not all who use hypnosis use hypnotizability scales. However, *Standards of Training in Clinical Hypnosis* (a volume devoted to requirements for the American Society of Clinical Hypnosis Certification in Clinical Hypnosis) recommends an awareness of hypnotic susceptibility scales such as the HIP (Hammond & Elkins, 1994). It is recommended that students appreciate that formal measurement scales provide objective methods of evaluating responsibility to hypnosis and who may be more likely to derive benefit from hypnotic techniques. The "Recommended Learning Objectives" referred to are:

A.  Demonstrate awareness of the advantages and the limitations or disadvantages in using formal measures of hypnotic responsibility.

B.  Identify the most commonly used hypnotic susceptibility scales (Hammond & Elkins, 1994).

Most formal hypnotic measurement scales take approximately an hour to be completed. The HIP was devised to fill a need for a shorter test for hypnotizability. The short time this test takes (six or so minutes) is much more practical for the busy therapist.

The following list of 11 reasons for using the HIP was developed by Dr. Fraser:

1.  ***The Hypnotic Induction Profile introduces hypnosis without pressure to have a formal hypnotic experience***
    The thought of "being put under" hypnosis may cause anxiety for some. However to undergo a brief clinical assessment for hypnotic *capacity* during which the individual is aware of what is happening serves as a gentle introduction to hypnosis before a formal hypnotic intervention. The emphasis is on assessment rather than being hypnotized.

2.  ***Testing raises professional acceptability***
    A test that produces an assessment scale may be more acceptable to colleagues who do not use hypnosis. It takes away much of the mystery and skepticism surrounding hypnosis (if there is a test, there must be something to test).

3.  ***It is a quick estimate of hypnotic rapport***
    In the approximately six minutes it takes for testing and scoring, the therapist can gauge rapport by the ease of compliance to the directions given during the testing. On the other hand, noncompliance during the testing or difficulties in following directions may portend impediments to the use of hypnosis, i.e., lack of hypnotic capacity, trust issues, fear of hypnosis, or cognitive impairment.

4. **Safely models the induction technique**

Having successfully done the HIP assessment, subjects feel more comfortable in agreeing to an induction strategy based on what they have already experienced.

5. **Dispels the myth of loss of control and loss of awareness when hypnotized**

Experiencing hypnotic phenomena during the HIP testing, and being able to still speak to the therapist and recall the majority, if not all of the testing, allows a cognitive reappraisal of hypnosis as being safer than the subject might have thought.

6. **A "user-friendly" six-minute estimate of hypnotic capacity**

The HIP is engaging and light, i.e., having subject make an arm float through imagery. This is non-threatening and often invokes smiles, easing any preconceived anxiety. This gentle approach generally enhances the rapport between therapist and subject.

7. **HIP can act as a differential test**

In conversation disorders, for instance, one would generally expect a high hypnotic induction profile. A subject with a low profile would more likely set off an alarm concerning such a diagnosis (of course, a high profile would not equal confirmation of such a diagnosis, even though it would be more compatible with such a diagnosis).

8. **May uncover "compensated" neurological conditions**

Although uncommon, this writer has used the HIP in referrals for conversion disorders. For example, a patient was referred to see if an upper limb tremor was psychogenic. With arm levitation instructions in the HIP the tremor became quite a bit worse. This response signaled that the condition was probably organic, i.e., the subject had over time likely compensated for the neurologic difficulties dampening down the tremor. With the HIP testing, this compensation was bypassed. Indeed, a MRI two weeks later confirmed a neurological disorder and the question of conversion disorder was dropped. The HIP had alerted us to this possibility before the MRI evidence was provided. In addition, the subject only scored in the midrange of the HIP.

9. **The HIP has internal checks and balances**

A person with a high eye-roll profile would generally have a high induction score. When these are vastly different, it may be a sign of subject noncooperation (i.e., eye roll, 0/10 in induction) or unconscious resistance.

10. ***Ease of referral to other therapists***
    Being able to refer a subject to a colleague and pass on a clinical scale such as "eye-roll profile 4/4, induction score 0/16" provides more clinical information than a statement such as, "I have used hypnosis with this subject."

11. ***This writer believes that no other six-minute noninvasive clinical tests in the fields of psychiatry and psychology provide so much clinical information***
    This writer used the HIP only once with each patient and subsequently uses a modified abbreviated induction based on the HIP. All patients with whom hypnosis is to be employed are first given the HIP. The HIP may also be used alone for diagnostic purposes as in assessment of conversion disorders or dissociative disorders but generally hypnosis would also be used clinically in the latter.

## *Dr. Spiegel introduces three basic components of the HIP*

1. The eye roll, as a biological measurement that records presumed biological trance capacity.

2. Subjective reports by the subject of hypnotic experience, including dissociation, involuntariness, and sensory alteration.

3. Behavioral change, including response to a challenge of arm levitation and response to a cut-off signal ending the hypnotic experience. "The HIP is both a procedure for trance induction and a disciplined measure of hypnotic capacity standardized on a patient population in a clinical setting" (Spiegel & Spiegel, 2004).

# *Measuring the Hypnotic Induction Profile*

## *Up-gaze*

Get as comfortable as possible with your arms resting on the arms of the chair and both feet up. Now look toward me. As you hold your head in that position, look up toward your eyebrows – now toward the top of your head.

**UP-GAZE:** 0–1–2–3–4

Measuring the amount of sclera rising from below.

Up-gaze can be scored 0, 1, 2, 3, or 4, according to Figure 1:

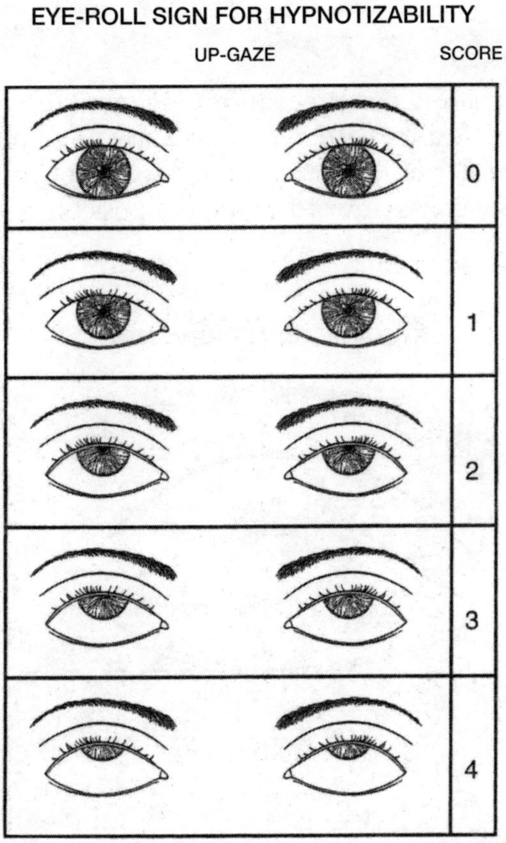

**EYE-ROLL SIGN FOR HYPNOTIZABILITY**

UP-GAZE                                          SCORE

*Figure 1*

- Score 0 when there is no sclera between the two borders.
- Score 1 for any amount of sclera, however small, between the two borders.
- Score 2 when the distance falls below or approximately on the midline of the eye.

Midline is an imaginary horizontal center that runs between the inner and outer corners of the eye.

- Score 3 when the amount of sclera reaches a little above the imaginary midline.
- Score 4 when the amount of sclera rises far above the midlines.

## Eye Roll

As you continue to look upward, close your eyelids slowly. That's right close, close, close…

**ROLL:** 0–1–2–3–4

The eye roll begins the induction procedure and is an important part of the profile grade. The eye roll is a measure of the distance, or amount of visible sclera between the lower border of the iris and the lower eyelid, exhibited when the subject simultaneously gazes upward as high as possible and slowly closes the eyelids (Figure 2).

### EYE-ROLL MEASUREMENT

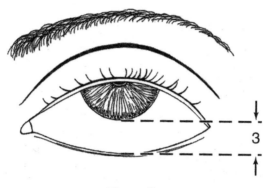

*Figure 2*

As the eyes are closing, score 0, 1, 2, 3, or 4.

- Score 0 when there is no sclera between the two borders.
- Score 1 for any amount of sclera, however small, between the two borders.
- Score 2 when the distance falls below or approximately on the midline of the eye.

Midline is an imaginary horizontal center that runs between the inner and outer corners of the eye.

- Score 3 when the amount of sclera reaches a little above the imaginary midline.
- Score 4 when the amount of sclera rises far above the midlines.

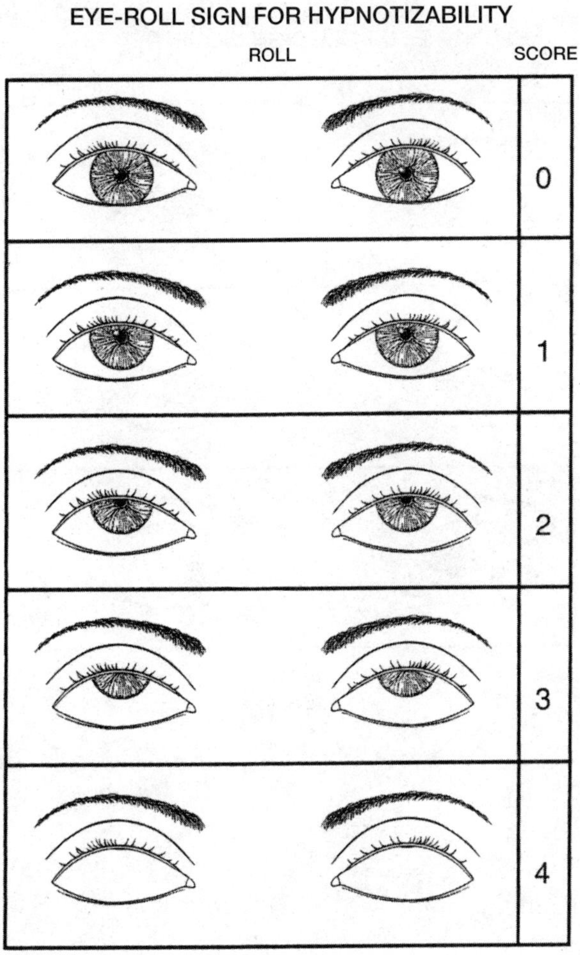

**EYE-ROLL SIGN FOR HYPNOTIZABILITY**

*Figure 3*

## Squint

**SQUINT:** 0–1–2–3–4

The eye-roll sign is part of the HIP scoring procedure only. It includes the procedures for items Roll and Squint (see Figure 4).

Our hypothesis is that the eye-roll sign, a measurement of mobility in extraocular eye movements, taps inherent potential capacity for experiencing hypnosis. It is part of the profile grade. The sign consists of the roll and squint measurements added together. Most often, though, a roll with no squint is found. It is sometimes observed that the score for the eye-roll sign remains stable and the scores for its two components vary (e.g., on the first examination, a subject shows a 2 roll and a 1 squint; the next examination, the person shows a 1 roll and a 2 squint). The eye-roll sign does not change over time for a given subject.

**EYE-ROLL SIGN (SQUINT)**

SCORE

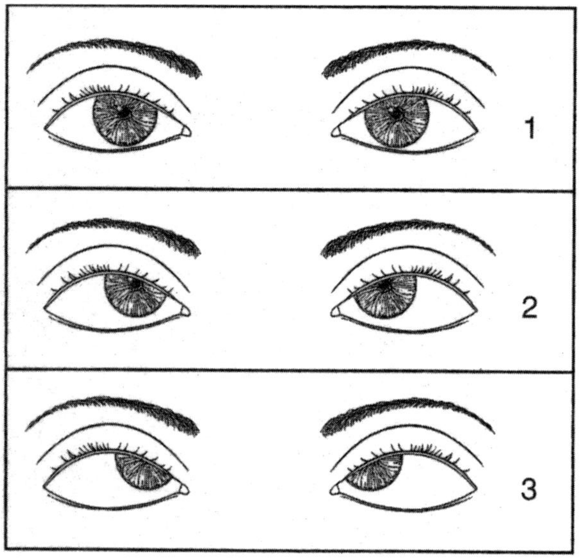


*Figure 4*

# Hypnotic Induction Profile
## Evaluation Sheet

Name _____ Date _____

Age _____ Sequence _____ Initial _____ Previous ___ When _____

Position of Subject:  Chair–Stool ❏   Supine ❏   Chair ❏   Standing ❏

**Item**

| | | |
|---|---|---|
| A _____ | Up-Gaze | 0 – 1 – 2 – 3 – 4 |
| B _____ | Roll: | 0 – 1 – 2 – 3 – 4 |
| C _____ | Squint: | 0 – 1 – 2 – 3 |
| D _____ | Eye-Roll Sign (roll + squint) | 0 – 1 – 2 – 3 – 4 |
| E _____ (× 1/2) | L. arm levitation instruction | 0 – 1 – 2 – 3 – 4 |
| F _____ | Comfortable  Tingle _____ | |
| G _____ | Dissociation | 0 –      – 1 – 2 |

H _____ Levitation

(Postinduction):
- no reinforcement 3 – 4
- 1st reinforcement 2 – 3
- 2nd reinforcement 1 – 2
- 3rd reinforcement 1
- 4th reinforcement 0 –

| | | |
|---|---|---|
| I _____ | Control Differential | 0 –    – 1 – 2 |
| J _____ | Cut-Off | 0 – |
| K _____ | Amnesia to Cut-off or No-Test | 0 –    – 1 – 2 |
| L _____ | Floating Sensation | 0 –    – 1 – 2 |

**Summary**

_____ Induction Score   Profile Grade 0 – 1 – 2 – 3 – 4 – 5

_____ Soft   _____ Zero   _____ Intact

_____ Minutes   _____ Decrement

_____ Special Zero   _____ Increment

In summary, a Hypnotic Induction Profile is an easily applied brief clinical measure of trance capacity. Although the HIP needs only be measured once, the instructions for it may also serve as an induction strategy for self-hypnosis and in further therapy sessions. Even if those employing hypnosis do not use hypnotic susceptibility scales, it is recommended that they be familiar with such scales. More measurement details can be found in *Trance and Treatment* (Spiegel & Spiegel, 2004).

An editorial in the *American Journal of Clinical Hypnosis* by Thurman Mott (2004) states: "Often there is no mention or instruction in assessing hypnotizability in clinical workshops or courses in hypnosis. This leaves the students with the impression that assessing hypnotizability is not important. It is my opinion that every basic workshop should teach the clinical assessment of hypnotizability by some method. Most of the reasons clinicians do not assess hypnotizability do not seem to apply to the nonobtrusive clinical assessment tools such as the HIP…" (p. 77).

# *References*

Hammond, D. C., & Elkins, G. R. (1994). *Standards of Training in Clinical Hypnosis,* (p. 10). Bloomingdale, IL: American Society of Clinical Hypnosis Press.

Mott, T. (2004). Assessing hypnotizability for case reports. *American Journal of Clinical Hypnosis,* 47(2), 77–78.

Spiegel H., & Spiegel, D. (2004). *Trance and Treatment: Clinical Uses of Hypnosis* (2nd edn), (p. 39). Arlington, VA: American Psychiatric Publishing, Inc.

## Chapter 4

# Mind/Body Communication

*Marlene E. Hunter*

In the past two decades, research has grown steadily to indicate the many ways in which mind and body communicate. Long gone are the days in which we thought that the brain was somehow an organ completely separate from the rest of the body. Instead, our knowledge of the intricacies of how the mind and the body communicate has grown by the proverbial leaps and bounds. This chapter puts some of these communication pathways into a more user-friendly perspective.

## What is "Mind"?

Is it the brain? No, not really. We can think of the brain as the universe within which "mind" operates. Part of that operation is the thinking process; part of it is the emotional process; and part of it is the way these processes affect the physiological responses within our bodies.

### The thinking process

"Thinking" involves neural pathways with the message traveling from one circuit of neurons to the next, and the next and so on. This involves the neuronal cells themselves, and the dendrites and axons that connect them.

But the thinking process is far more than that. We are wired, so to speak. I doubt that many of us think of the electric circuitry within us, but it is a crucial part of our whole. Think of energy, in this case, electrical energy, driving the machinery.

However, the second, equally crucial part of the mix includes all the biophysiological "juices," in other words the hormones and biochemicals providing the nutrient soup through which our brains and bodies can send messages from one part of us to another part of us.

## The emotional process

So what are "emotions"? They are responses to some trigger that is related to past experience, in other words, a memory. These responses in turn, elicit a response from the brain, involving the body's hormones and biochemicals. If this seems like a merry-go-round, that's because it is. The thinking process is really a body process and the emotional process is also a body process. And all of this contributes to the quintessential process of mind/body communication.

# What is "Body"?

We could think of "Body" as a collection of amino acids and fat, gussied up with some sinewy tissue and chunks of calcium, bathed in biophysiological juices and held together by a thin covering. The whole thing is interlaced with nerves. It sounds like the "Mind," minus, perhaps, the chunks of calcium (unless you count hardening of the arteries).

In fact, there is no way to separate mind and body. "Body memories" are reflections of extreme stress from the past. Insulin-producing cells can be found in the gut. Flashbacks, a specific kind of memory and therefore surely of the mind, produce the same physiological response in the body (shaking, sweating, tachycardia) as did the original episode.

These are just small examples of the various ways in which our minds and bodies communicate. The language has been a little tongue-in-cheek, but what follows will conform more to the sedate vocabulary of science.

# Mind/Body Communication

This is how I describe mind/body communication to my patients:

*A message comes into our awareness. It could come through what we see, or what we hear, what we might smell or taste or touch – in fact, through any of the senses. Whichever the route, the message triggers a memory.*

*The message passes from one set of neurons to the next, and the next, through the layers of the conscious mind, and continues into the subconscious mind, often finding a resting place in a small collection of neuronal circuits called the limbic system, deep in the right orbitofrontal cortex.*

*Once there, the message meets up with a plethora of other information. This "other information" might have to do with state-dependent learning, i.e., the emotional state that we are in when we devise (often subconsciously) a way to deal with the situation that will predicate how we will probably respond to a similar situation in the future; or to other experiences of which the memories linger, but more in the subconscious than the conscious. Or it might have to do with the psychosocial components of the situation, or even the environment.*

*Any or all of these could modify the message before it is sent further on in its journey.*

*The modified message proceeds through the hypothalamus, the "oldest" part of the brain in terms of evolution. I prefer to describe it as the most mature part of the brain. It continues to the brain stem, where it soon becomes juxtaposed near the pituitary gland, and it is sent to that tiny but incredibly important physiological entity by biochemical messenger.*

*The pituitary gland is, in a way, the grandfather gland in the body. It sends out hormones to prompt all the endocrine glands, and through some sort of internal intelligence it chooses which gland needs to be alerted. Perhaps it is the adrenals, so that they can in turn send out the "fight or flight" response hormones; or perhaps the thyroid gland, or the ovaries or testicles of the reproductive system.*

*These glands in turn send out their hormones, to stimulate the target organs and physiological systems in the body – heart, lungs, muscles or whatever the situation demands.*

*Then, the body, again in turn, sends the appropriate response back to the limbic system, where it might stay, becoming part of that huge subconscious memory bank, or continue further up the chain into the conscious, language-and-logic part of the brain and cognitive memory.*

I have explained this to hundreds of patients, in exactly this way, and have yet to find a situation in which the patient did not understand what I was talking about. Often, I will explain it when the patient is in hypnosis, but not always. It provides a kind of internal forum, wherein experience and memory may begin to link up and make sense where it had previously been inexplicable. This pathway is described visually in the chart overleaf.

## The Role of Memory

We remember things that we do not know that we are remembering. Often, we remember things differently from what actually happened. This often has to do with the emotional climate, or one's age, at the time of the experience. At times, we do not know that we have remembered something, and might never know

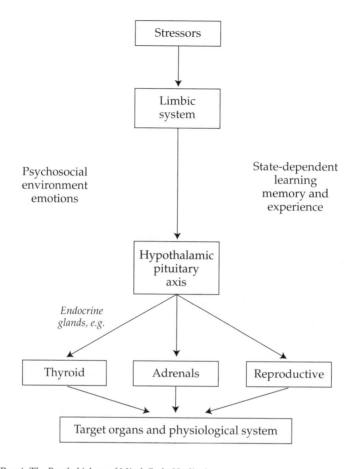

(Adapted from Rossi, *The Psychobiology of Mind–Body Healing*)

it, or it may surface in an entirely unexpected and/or intrusive way. There are two major types of memory: implicit and explicit.

## Implicit memory

"Implicit" memory could be called subconscious, or experiential, memory. It has four main factors:

- It is present at birth, or before birth
- It is behavioral, perceptual, emotional, somatosensory memory
- Focal attention is not required for encoding
- Attachment experiences become *encoded* and *reinforced* deep within the brain.

An example of implicit memory being present at (or before) birth would be a howling infant, newborn, being put onto his or her mother's chest and settling down immediately, because the baby hears the mother's heartbeat, which he or she has been listening to in the womb for many months.

As stated, it is *experiential* in nature. It is memory of something that we have experienced, not read about or discovered in some cognitive manner.

"Somatosensory" memory is the basis for what are more commonly called "body memories." These were denied for decades as being imaginary, but there is nothing imaginary about them, and they are linked to past experience which are important factors in some of the difficult chronic syndromes, such as chronic fatigue syndrome or chronic pain syndromes, for which no apparent reason can be found. The literature on these research studies can easily be found on the Web.

Flashbacks may also fall into this category, as the person having the flashback has been catapulted into the past, not remembering, in the sense of knowing where he or she is and realizing that this is a memory of something that happened, but simultaneously *being right back there again*, with all the sights, smells, noise and chaos that were part of the original experience. Just ask any war veteran.

"Focal attention is not required for encoding" refers to the fact that these memories were not cognitive, but rather what the person was experiencing at the time making a searing impact on the subconscious mind.

"Attachment experiences" have to do with a very young child having, or not having, someone in his or her life for whom trust and dependability are foremost. Indeed, it is the way we learn how to trust, and we learn it from someone who knows how to trust. If there, it blossoms into being able to trust others (and recognizing the warning signals if that other person is untrustworthy), and also being able to trust oneself. Attachment disorders, as they are called, have secured a position front and center in the psychology and psychotherapy fields. Implicit memory plays a huge role in mind/body communication, because it is without words, until and unless we put it into words at which time it can become explicit memory.

## Explicit memory

"Explicit" implies that we can put words to the memory. It develops through conscious awareness. It is semantic and autobiographical. Focal attention is required for encoding. Hippocampal processing is required for storage. Selected events become part of permanent memory (cortical consolidation). It is *narrative* memory.

The relationship between mind/body communication and explicit memory is not nearly as profound as is that between implicit memory and mind/body communication. Of course, there are connections nonetheless, but the profundity is much less (Siegel, 1999).

## Hypnosis and Mind/Body Communication

These descriptions of implicit and explicit memory become more important if we are to utilize memory as a therapeutic tool. Because it is the mind/body connection that is paramount in such endeavors, we rely on implicit memory as a pathway to the hypnotic link when looking for relief from distressing symptoms.

I simply teach the following mantra-like requests for the subconscious to be an active part of the healing process:

> *Let my subconscious mind and my body, communicate*
> *Each giving the other – mind giving body, body giving mind*
> *The information that each needs*
> *So that together, they can continue to collaborate and cooperate*
> *Towards the achievement of the goal.*

There is therefore a very simple post-hypnotic suggestion that can go along with this: Mind/Body Communication, Collaboration, Cooperation (MB/CCC). I suggest that the person say that to him- or herself, aloud or silently, or read it or write it, or sing it several times a day.

This should be accompanied by an *image* of what the goal might be. It doesn't matter what the image is, whether it makes sense to anybody else or not. It is important because it *is* an image, and the language of the subconscious mind is imagery, not words. This simple recipe is the essence of mind/body communication, and it works.

## Stress and the Brain

Because stress affects the brain at the subconscious level, even more than the conscious level, it is important to say a few words about it. Stress plays a major role in implicit memory. Remember that stress is not necessarily bad, it simply makes an impact. Nevertheless, negative stressors are a huge part of such things as post-traumatic stress disorder, the dissociative disorders and other trauma-related dysfunctions.

Our brains can be, and often are, sensitized in various ways. The sensitization of the brain is known as *use-dependent development*. The brain is designed to adjust to its chemistry and electrical circuitry to meet the demands of the environment. Experience determines which circuits of neurons become activated and join other circuits of neurons. Circuits that are repeatedly activated *(positively or negatively)* are *strengthened* and *stabilized*, and can be turned on with less and less stimulation *(positive or negative)*.

Parts of the brain mature at different ages and stages of the person. How those parts work together depends on the experiences to which the child is exposed *(positively or negatively)* (Siegel, 1999).

It is easy to see the role that sensitization can play in the mind/body communication spectrum. Sadly, it is an aspect that people often neglect to recognize, or at least do not fully recognize its importance. Because of the time span involved, usually from early infancy to teens, the brain is incredibly vulnerable to such sensitization, and that vulnerability can be paramount in such problems as post-traumatic stress disorder.

It is also very important when working with the chronic syndromes – chronic pain, irritable bowel disease, chronic fatigue and so on. It is the body, complaining and wanting to be heard.

Extreme stress "shuts down" the thinking brain, especially the language and logic areas of the left hemisphere. This "short-circuits" the cognitive system, leaving only the autonomic reactions of the stress response.

| STRESS MECHANISM | DEFENSE MECHANISM |
|---|---|
| *Freeze* | *Dissociate* |
| | Project, Displacement |
| *Flee* | Denial, Rationalization |
| | Distortion, etc. |
| *Fight* | |

Powerful emotions, generated in the *right* hemisphere, cannot be processed in the *left*, cognitive hemisphere (no language). Stress (chronic, severe) inhibits the flow of information within the brain, and between brain and body (Siegel, 1999).

We see, again, the huge role that mind/body communication can, and does, play in our health, both mental and physical. Unfortunately, there is still this tendency to think of this delicate and crucial mechanism as something imagined or deliberately made up in order to get attention. There is nothing to be welcomed in the chronic syndromes, in sexual dysfunction, in panic and anxiety attacks. People need to learn ways with which the impact of these conditions can be minimized.

So the question becomes … *Can we "think"' ourselves into better physical and mental health? If so, then how?* The obvious answers would be hypnosis, or meditation, or mindfulness, or yoga, or simply bull-headed determination, but let us always remember the Mind/Body Communication Triangle:

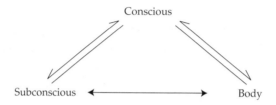

Communication goes back and forth along all sides of this triangle, all the time, in both directions, but it is at its strongest, and most important, along the base of the triangle, between the subconscious and the body.

We can facilitate this with hypnosis:

- To improve mind/body communication
- Visualization
- Taste, touch, aroma, sound – involving all the senses
- Push the pause button (a way to give a little break when things become overwhelming)
- Push the replay button (ready to tackle it gain)
- Self-talk

## *Metaphors*

Metaphors are simply hypnotic inductions under another name. It doesn't really matter whether the person is in a recognized state of hypnosis or not as the results are the same.

The only rule is that the metaphor must be relevant to the patient. It is a way to avoid formal hypnosis, for someone who is uncomfortable with the idea of going into a trance state (perceived as being out of control).

One of my favorite metaphors is the "Pool of Resources." It goes like this:

*Imagine yourself in a desert. There is an oasis up ahead that you can just see. When you reach the oasis, there is pool there, and the water in the pool is clean, clear and cool.*

*You look around to find a river of some sort, feeding the pool, but you cannot find one. That is because it is an* underground river *that is feeding the pool, such as is often found in such circumstances. Consequently, the pool is constantly renewed and refreshed.*

*We also have a Pool of Resources, deep within us. It is constantly renewed and refreshed by the underground river of the subconscious mind. Everything that happens to us, and how we* respond *to everything that happens to us, adds to the river and therefore to the Pool of Resources.*

*We may, if we realize that we have been in a similar situation before, swear that we will never go that way again. However, we may also say that we could explore some ways of adapting what went well in the earlier situation, to the present situation; or, if the earlier situation was very positive, we might very well choose to do it again.*

*You have such Pool of Resources deep within you. It is always there, because it is within.*

*We may choose, at times, to give away something that comes from within – love, for example; at times, we may throw away something that comes from within; but no one can ever take away something that comes from within. The Pool of Resources is yours. It belongs to you.*

You may adapt this script to suit you and your patients. It can be very useful in bolstering that sense of self-worth that is so critical to each one of us, and which so many of those who come for help sadly lack.

Realistically, we are dealing with human nature. What is possible may not be probable, and vice versa. But then … so what? The connections are there. We need to appreciate them as well as utilize them. Mind/body communication, collaboration, cooperation – it works.

# References

Rossi, E. L. (1986). *The Psychobiology of Mind–body Healing: New Concepts of Therapeutic Hypnosis.* New York: Norton.

Siegel, D. (1999). *The Developing Mind: Toward a Neurobiology of Interpersonal Experience.* New York: Guilford.

# Chapter 5

# Psychosomatic Medicine

*Marlene E. Hunter*

## What is "psychosomatic medicine"?

For hundreds of years, in the Western world, we have thought of medical problems as being distinct from emotional problems. One of the pioneers in challenging this concept was Hans Selye, a Canadian physician, who spoke openly about his belief that stress was a significant factor in many of our physical problems.

However, it was with the publication of *Psychoneuroimmunology*, edited by Robert Ader in 1981, that the medical world began to give real credence to what we now consider indisputable: that mind and body are irrevocably linked and our health, in every respect, depends on both healthy minds and healthy bodies.

Earlier in this medical revolution, Franz Alexander had related seven conditions as belonging to this new concept: essential hypertension, peptic ulcer, ulcerative colitis, hyperthyroidism, regional enteritis, rheumatoid arthritis and bronchial asthma (Alexander, 1950). I have always found it amusing that three of the seven are connected to the digestive system – what one might call a "gut reaction." I apologize for the bad pun, but not for the awareness of the link.

The word *psychosomatic* comes from the two roots, "psyche," meaning mind, and "soma," meaning body. When it first came into medical jargon, it was considered just that – jargon: another way of implying "imaginary." However, Ader's book brought clearer focus, and the dawning realization that we are never disconnected at the neck and that what happens in our emotional world has an impact on our physiological world, and vice versa.

We could easily think of various contributions from the psyche:

Anger, fear, trust/distrust, anxiety, love/hate

Just as easily can we think of the role of the soma:

The neuroendophysiological and biochemical responses to the emotions

# What is "behavioral medicine"?

This term implies that we can help people improve their health by showing them ways to modify their behavior.

Implicit in this concept is that the person wants to and is ready to work to effect those changes. As clinicians, that is a factor that we must never ignore.

Viewed from these perspectives, it is easy to acknowledge that *everything* is psychosomatic. True, some things are more psyche and some are more soma, but "you can't have one without the other," as the old song says.

## Examples of conditions with psychogenic roots:

- Insomnia
- Panic attacks
- Being "stressed out"
- Inability to concentrate
- Nightmares

## Examples of conditions with somatogenic roots:

- Biochemical imbalance
- Hormonal deficiencies or excesses
- Infections
- Neoplasms
- Degenerative diseases: of the body and of the brain

# How do psychosomatic and behavioral concepts and approaches work together?

When we acknowledge that *everything is psychosomatic*, we are already in the realm of behavioral medicine. When we help people to shift or change their thinking and emotional response by changing their behavior, for example, this addresses the "psyche" directly, and therefore, secondly, affects the soma also.

One author who contributed significantly to these ideas is Ernest Rossi. In his book, *The Psychobiology of Mind–Body Healing*, published in 1986, he describes in great detail the mutual contributions of the brain, its hormones and biochemicals, and their demand for the body in turn to respond with its own hormones and biochemicals, which further affect the organs in the body. The body then responds, sends its own messages back to the brain, and the process is repeated. It is the quintessential biofeedback mechanism.

Further information came to the world's awareness through the works of Candace Pert, Robert Sapolsky and others throughout the next two decades.

## Getting the data, so that the process can begin

As physicians, psychologists, therapists, nurses and others in the field, our first task is to identify the patient's beliefs and needs in light of his or her past experiences.

We do this, of course, by taking a very careful history, listening with our eyes as well as out ears, paying attention to voice inflections, facial expression, body language and emotional tone/expression.

Among the important questions, we ask: "What were you *told* when it began? How did you *interpret* that? *Who was it* who told you that? How did you *feel* when he/she told you that?"

There are clues to be found in each and every question and answer, and they are crucial if we are to be able to help the patient to the best of our abilities.

It is also important to understand the situation in which patients heard these early questions, and to ascertain their emotional and physical state at the time.

## Some techniques

There are hundreds of techniques that are helpful in these situations. However, we are specifically concerned, here, with hypnotic approaches, so we need to search, pick and choose those with which we feel comfortable – and also to develop our own. The following are some that I have found very helpful over the years. Readers may feel free to take them and amend them as their own.

Remember that patients/clients are already in a state of eyes-open hypnosis as soon as they enter our offices, the emergency room, the case room, the dentist's office or other such setting. Think of the five basic qualities of hypnosis:

- Decrease in global awareness
- Inward focusing
- Economy of movement
- Tendency to take things personally and literally
- Tendency to ignore "no" and its correlates.

I have just described a person in hypnosis, but I have also just described someone who is in a state of stress, simply by being where he or she is and for whatever the reason is behind the visit. It is more useful, then, to communicate with patients/clients as if they were in a trance (which they are).

## *(1) Break the Pattern*

This is a very simple technique that works well when the patient is, first of all, able to recognize that there *is* a pattern to the behavior, and secondly that the behavior is a response predicated on his or her interpretation of the situation.

In hypnosis, ask the patient to recognize both the behavior and response, and to do that meticulously, recognizing every detail. This is important, because it is some detail of the person's choosing that provides the first link in the chain to be broken. It works best to start with something very small, some minor modification that the patient/client can, and is willing at that time, to make.

Point out that in any system, when one thing changes (no matter how small a change), everything else has to shuffle around to accommodate the change, and that as soon as that begins to happen, the whole situation changes, too.

Once the process is underway, it continues on its own steam and at its own pace until the situation is resolved and/or a new way of responding is created.

## *(2) Trigger Curiosity*

While he or she is in hypnosis, invite the patient to be curious about some aspect of the situation – why it began, for example, or what has kept it going, or what did this situation add in terms of day-to-day living.

Then invite him or her to be curious as to what it would be like *without* this particular aspect, and encourage some hypnotic exploration into a future where it has changed. If the patient chooses to do that, then suggest that he or she ask that the mind and the body, *together*, do whatever needs to be done to begin such a change in that particular aspect.

By implying that it is not necessary to change everything, the patient is more comfortable than he or she would be with the scary thought that the whole thing is going to turn upside down.

## (3) Thank the Protector

One of the most useful hypnotic techniques that I have found, and one that can be applied to many, many situations, is the idea that the subconscious is one's most fierce protector, and that all responses to situations begin as a way to protect the system from unknown onslaughts. This includes habits, of course, as well as emotional responses.

The problem lies in the fact that after a while the "protection" has become an intrusion or a hindrance, but the good old subconscious is still trying valiantly to protect it.

The technique for easing this dilemma is very simple: while in hypnosis, invite the patient to say "Thank you" to the Protector for the *intention* to protect, recognizing that at one time it was a very important help and support, but that now, the situation/life circumstances are different, and a new way needs to be found to take care of the present challenges.

Usually this takes some time, and should be repeated frequently over the next few days or weeks, but after a while one notices little shifts. Remember to thank the Protector for the little shifts!

## (4) Get to Know the Saboteur(s)

This may be for the more sophisticated patient, but it works.

Almost always, an apparent saboteur in one's subconscious is really an upside-down Protector. I usually use an example from one of my dissociative patients who had an ego state whose job it was to "take care of the snakes." Snakes had been part of this patient's early childhood abuse. Over a long period of time I was allowed to get to know the Snake-keeper and we worked out a compromise.

All went very well for several months, until the day the patient turned up, white as a ghost, and said, "The snakes are back."

I asked to speak to the Snake-keeper who, much to my relief condescended to come to speak with me. When I asked her to explain the situation, she hissed (yes, hissed) that the woman "*…was talking too much, of course!*"

Of course. During her childhood, if she tried to tell what was happening to her, she was abused and punished more. The Snake-keeper was afraid I would do the same thing. It was her way of keeping the child (now a woman) safe.

So, sometimes, getting to know the Saboteur, i.e., the part of the person's subconscious that appears to be sabotaging the person's efforts to change, and who is really trying to protect him or her from a misperceived danger, can change the situation for the better. Offering careful hypnotic suggestions to clarify that now there is no danger is the way to go.

Notice the similarities in this situation and the one above it: Saboteurs are upside-down Protectors. *Parts therapy*

## (5) Back to Before

It may be useful for the patient, in hypnosis, to travel backwards in time to the time before the particular problem was there. This is also a technique for the more experienced patient.

Once back to the time before the problem existed, the subconscious is invited to begin coming forward in time again, but this time and any time, it encountered any factor that would be a contributor to the eventual dysfunction, the subconscious and the body *together* did whatever had to be done to take care of that danger before it even started.

Explain that no one knows how long that process will take, but it will just keep on at its own pace until the "present present" (as opposed to the "past present" or "future present") is reached. It may take minutes, hours or days. One can have confidence in the subconscious.

## (6) Rehearse Successful Recovery

With this technique, the person goes into the "future present," to the time when all relief, healing, adjustments and so forth, have already been made and life has been rewarding for a long time.

Enjoy that happy state.

Then slowly begin coming *backwards in time toward the present,* paying attention to all the road signs along the way so that, when the person makes that journey chronologically, his or her subconscious will recognize the signs and keep the person on the right track.

## (7) Cognitive Adaptations

Perhaps surprisingly, one can utilize the hypnotic state to access cognitive means of adaptation.

This can also be done without using hypnosis (although, again, while in the therapist's office, the patient is already in an altered state of consciousness). Some people respond extremely well to a cognitive approach, perhaps even better than to the hypnotic approach.

It takes time and considerable energy to sit with the patient and thoroughly discuss the situation from a conscious, logical aspect and help him or her to perceive a new pattern of mind/body interaction.

## (8) State-Dependent Learning

In simple terms, state-dependent learning refers to the tendency the mind has to continue to respond in the same way as before to a similar situation.

It is upfront when there has been trauma, and the victim has had to find a way to survive. It's not hard to understand why the subconscious wants to use what works, over and over again. The fact that it worked before, but may not work now, is at the conscious, logical level but not in the experiential memory banks of the limbic system.

If this is explored in hypnosis, is must be done with great finesse and respect. Remember that the subconscious is extremely protective and very, very suspicious.

Just understanding about state-dependent learning is helpful to one who has had trauma in his or her life, or has come, usually subconsciously, to the belief that the present response is useful.

## (9) Affirmations

Good old affirmations can always have a useful role to play.

It should be remembered that, for our purposes, an affirmation is a statement about the future, made in the present tense, as if it has already happened in the past (thus a nice juxtaposition and interaction of time past, time present and time future). An easy example is, "It feels wonderful to be well again."

This utilization of tense changes is far more effective than something like the old adage, "Every day, in every way, I'm getting better and better." It relies on hope, rather than stating a fait accompli.

## (10) Others

Techniques such as working with "the past belongs to the past" or inviting the adult to go back to help the inner child deal with a situation are also useful.

Many patients respond well to exploring the actual relationship in their individual situations of psyche versus soma. If this is the case, one can, if suitable, utilize hypnotic techniques to help establish useful pathways towards change.

Through these various techniques – and there are many, many more – we are helping our patients to understand the mind/body connection and thus, the huge role that psychosomatic and behavioral medicine plays in our lives and in theirs.

## *References*

Ader, R. (Ed.) (1981). *Psychoneuroimmunology*. New York: Academic Press.
Alexander, F. (1950). *Psychosomatic Medicine*. New York: Norton.
Pert, C. (1986). Emotions in body, not just in brain. *Brain/Mind Bulletin*, 11(4), 1.
Rossi, E. (1986). *The Psychobiology of Mind–Body Healing*. New York: Norton.
Selye, H. (1974). *Stress Without Distress*. New York: Signet.

# Part II
# *Dental Hypnosis*

# Chapter 6

# *Rapid Relaxation*

## *The Practical Management of Pre-Op Anxiety*

*John G. Lovas and David A. Lovas*

## *Introduction*

Dental anxiety or phobia is a common and challenging disorder for both patients and practitioners. The prevalence of dental anxiety ranges from 4 to 20% (Milgrom, Fiset, Melnick, & Weinstein, 1988) and it has been shown to have a negative impact on dental health (Vassend, 1993). Moreover, data suggest that many dentists have difficulty both identifying dental anxiety (Baron, Logan, & Kao, 1990) and treating it effectively (Moore & Brodsgaard, 2001). Fortunately, there is considerable evidence supporting the use of behavioral interventions for lessening patient anxiety (Kvale, Berggre, & Milgrom, 2004) and possibly mitigating practitioner-stress experienced in the modern, fast-paced dental practice.

Severe dental phobics avoid dental encounters until advanced dental disease necessitates emergency treatment, usually under general anesthetic. Those with less severe dental anxiety can usually be managed with sedative pharmacologic agents, administered via intravenous, oral, or inhalation routes (Dionne & Kaneko, 2002). Formal hypnosis is another effective, though underutilized, method for managing dental anxiety (Thompson, 1997; Hermes, Truebger, Hakim, & Seig, 2005).

The vast majority of dental patients are treated without any formal attempt to manage fear and anxiety. Yet, it is known that pre- and intra-operative stress, elicits the stereotypical "stress response" or "fight-or-flight" response, characterized by increased sympathetic, as well as central nervous system arousal, most clearly manifested by increased heart rate, diaphoresis, and increased skeletal muscle activity (Lundgren, Berggren, & Carlsson, 2001). Immediately prior to receiving local anesthetic, "unmanaged" patients usually display overt signs of stress: changed facial expression (e.g., frown); tensing of muscle groups (e.g., gripping the armrest); and abnormal breathing (rapid shallow breathing or holding the breath). Of the minority who appear outwardly calm, most on direct questioning will readily admit to some apprehension.

How can we help the majority of our dental patients better manage their immediate pre-op mild-to-moderate anxiety? Although effective communication, persuasive ability, and behavior management are recognized as essential foundations of ideal patient management (Hosey, 2002), these topics are rarely dealt with in any depth in dental or medical schools, where the overwhelming emphasis is on pharmacological approaches (Bub, 2006).

Do noninvasive relaxation techniques have proven benefits over the status quo? Recent studies in other disciplines examining the effect of relaxation techniques on post-operative pain and narcotic use have shown mixed results. However, consistently positive outcomes have been demonstrated in the domains that are particularly pertinent for the preoperative dental patient – including anxiety, patient satisfaction, and so on (Gavin, Litt, Kahn, Onyiuke, & Kozol, 2006; Haase, Schwenk, Hermann, & Muller, 2005).

## *Hypnosis*

Hypnosis, the very essence of which is "good chair-side manner" – effective, empathic doctor–patient communication – is a unique "soft" technology. Before the advent of general anesthesia, hundreds of major surgeries were performed under hypnosis alone, effectively managing not only severe pre- and intra-op anxiety, but also severe intra-operative pain. A dramatic modern-day demonstration of this mostly forgotten potential for hypnosis was Dr. Rausch's carefully documented major abdominal surgery, performed without any drugs, using self-hypnosis alone (Rausch, 1980). Though clearly a powerful modality, with broad dental applications, and known to the dental profession for over 100 years, hypnosis remains underutilized. A good definition of hypnosis in this context is "a formalized method of applying the techniques of attention modification, paced breathing, and muscle relaxation" (Milgrom, 2002).

Barriers to its broader use include: the requirement for additional training, the need to obtain formal consent, the need for extra chair time, popular misconceptions (based on stage hypnotists) about the nature of clinical hypnosis, and finally, roughly a fifth of the population are unable to enter sufficiently profound trance states (Meechan, Robb, & Seymour, 1998). These barriers apply to formal hypnosis, but many useful elements of hypnosis can be adapted, and used informally to help ease dental fear and anxiety. Important core principles of hypnosis are listed in Hammond (Hammond, 1990):

1. First and foremost, establishing a warm, understanding, caring, cooperative, respectful relationship with the patient will reduce defensiveness and maximize effectiveness.

2. Creating "positive expectancy" by behaving and speaking confidently, like we fully expect our suggestions will occur, will inspire confidence in patients.

3. Emphasizing "imagination and imagery rather than appealing to the conscious will" circumvents "the law of reversed effect." The latter is based on the observation that the harder one consciously tries to do something, the more difficult it is to succeed; for example, trying to fall asleep.

4. Repeating a suggestion and concentrating repeatedly on a goal or idea increases the chance of success.

5. Patiently adjusting one's pace to the patient's rate of response ("principle of successive approximations"), yet retaining positive expectancy, increases success.

6. "The law of dominant effect" suggests that it is more effective to appeal to the patient's dominant emotion. The patient's anxiety can be resolved only by following the clinician's suggestions.

7. Linking the patient's motivations and goals with the clinician's suggestions is encouragement ("the carrot principle"), and less likely to be resisted and thus more effective than pushing the patient.

8. According to the "principle of positive suggestion," clinicians should focus on creating positive motivation and attitudes in patients rather than trying to override their existing motives or attitudes.

9. Giving the patient encouraging feedback ("principle of positive reinforcement"), during and after the session, catalyzes the entire experience.

10. Obtaining a series of yes responses from the patient creates an "acceptance set," that is, a state of mind in which it is very hard to disagree with the subsequent suggestions. Statements about universally experienced situations also elicit nonverbal yes responses.

In most forms of hypnosis, the clinician's tone of voice and body language are intentionally consistently soothing, monotonous, and congruent with the aim of relaxing and reassuring the patient. Great care is taken to choose words ("bit of discomfort" versus "pain") that are least anxiety-provoking. The fine points of communication employed in hypnosis (Graham, 1998) are equally useful clinically outside of formal hypnosis settings.

## *Meditation*

Attention modification and paying attention to one's breath are also the key elements of formal sitting meditation practice. The two most prevalent forms of meditation are concentration and mindfulness. Of the two, the concentration type is the simplest and most calming. In concentration meditation, attention is focused on a single object (e.g., one's own breath) to the exclusion of all other objects. As distracting thoughts or sensations arise, they are gently let go. Repeatedly, awareness is returned to the primary object of attention. As the mind stabilizes on this object, tranquility ensues (Olendzki, 2005). Attention to the breath in the base of the lungs stabilizes abdominal breathing, and elicits the relaxation response. Theoretically, abdominal breathing induces relaxation at least partially due to direct stimulation of the phrenic plexus of the parasympathetic nervous system.

Focusing detailed attention specifically on the physical sensation of the breath, first and foremost anchors the patient in the body, which is always in "real time," whereas anxiety is anticipatory, related to the fear of future events. Since (complete/detailed) attention can only be on one object at a time, anxiety-provoking thinking about the quality (e.g., excessive rate, ineffectiveness) of breathing is displaced. The patient is guided to experience "the visceral embodiedness of every moment" (Olendzki, 2006).

The US National Health Interview Survey 2002 revealed that of the 10 complementary and alternative medicine therapies most commonly used within the past 12 months, most were "mind–body" interventions: biofeedback, meditation, guided imagery, progressive relaxation, deep breathing exercises, hypnosis, yoga, tai chi, qi gong, and prayer for health reasons. They found that 10.2% of Americans have meditated, 14.6% have used deep breathing exercises, and 1.8% of Americans have had hypnosis. It is important to note that mind–body medicine is part of mainstream health care in sharp contrast to "alternative therapies," such as homeopathy, naturopathy, chelation therapy, and the like. Mind–body medicine's central tenet is that thoughts and emotions produce health effects. These are measurable physiologic changes, with a long history of scientific validation in peer-reviewed journals (Jacobs, 2001).

Barriers to practicing formal meditation include: inadequate knowledge about meditation; lack of time to practice; reluctance to "sit and do nothing"; the misperception that meditation entails abandoning one's own religion; and perhaps most important, reluctance to change one's current lifestyle.

# The Rapid Relaxation Method

Over the years, the senior author (JL) developed a practical preoperative anxiety management method by condensing the essential elements of hypnosis and meditation into a very brief set of instructions, called Rapid Relaxation (RR).

## Patient selection, indications, and contraindications

Clearly patients must be able to understand and follow instructions. A patient's frustration over inability to follow instructions can undermine the effects of the dentist's soothing voice.

This technique is ideal for that large majority of patients who typically undergo dental treatment without prior medication (anxiolytics, sedatives), yet suffer fear and anxiety pre- and intra-operatively. Clear signs of pre-op stress range from saying out loud, "I'm scared," to exhibiting pallor, clammy hands, rapid shallow respiration, rapid pulse, hands gripping each other or the armrest, etc. Even those who appear calm immediately before the dental procedure should be asked if they're anxious – often the response is affirmative.

A small proportion of the most frightened patients seem to ignore the RR instructions. Some appear too frightened to pay attention, and a few have stated that they opted to use their own coping strategy.

Instructions for RR are ideally given during the two or three minutes it takes to ensure profound topical anesthesia. The patient is recumbent in the dental chair, generally with a dental assistant helping, and sometimes one of the patient's relatives is also sitting near the patient. The following is the general procedure:

1.  Show the reassuringly soft, cotton-tipped topical anesthetic applicator to the patient, stating "This will first comfortably numb the surface." Apply and hold the topical anesthetic in place.

2.  Assess the patient's overall body language. If the hands are clasped together, often pressing down on the solar plexus area, or firmly gripping the armrest, suggest in a calm, slow, reassuring voice "You might find it more comfortable to let your arms rest loosely on the armrest." Selective, gentle

humor like, "Please be easy on our equipment," is sometimes appropriate to lighten the mood. If the legs are crossed over the ankles (some patients actually press the upper ankle down firmly on the one below), suggest, "You'll likely find it more comfortable uncrossing your legs." If the eyes are open, suggest, "You might find it more comfortable closing your eyes – whatever's more comfortable for you."

The assistant and dentist should periodically check the patient's body language. When a raised shoulder, frown on forehead, or "white knuckles" clasping the arms of the chair is observed, gently touch the area and gently remind the patient to relax it.

3.  "If you like, we'll show you how you can feel more relaxed. Scan your whole body, from head to toes, and look for any areas of tightness and tension in your muscles. As you know, this 'guarding' doesn't really help you. Tight muscles only make you tired and tense. You can just let your muscles relax. Let them go – just like when you're really tired and you finally lie down in bed and feel your whole body sink into the mattress – allow your body to sink into the chair – completely relaxed, soft, floppy, like a baby or a puppy."

It's important to note that no one ever refused to have these instructions, or complained that they were given them. The word "might" is used intentionally to maintain a permissive, rather than authoritarian, tone.

4.  "Now that your body is nice and relaxed, you might notice that your thoughts are zipping around a hundred miles an hour, worrying about the future – 'what if this, what if that.' You know that this doesn't help either. It just makes you tired and anxious. A much better thing to do with your attention is to let it rest.

"A good place to let your attention rest is on the gentle feel of your breath at the bottom of your lungs. Allow your attention to rest on the subtle feel of your breath in your belt area. Each part of the breath – beginning, middle, and end – feels subtly different, and every breath is slightly different. Let your attention rest on this subtle feeling."

If breathing is not reasonably slow and adequately abdominal, remind the patient: "There's no need to try to control the breathing in any way, just simply observe the subtle feel of the breath way down in your belt area. Breathing deep down to the base of your lungs is very efficient, so you can breathe much slower."

5.  "You'll notice your attention drifting back to worrying thoughts – that's normal. Gently, patiently, just keep bringing your attention back to the subtle feel of your breath in your belt area. Allow it to rest there peacefully."

6.  Shortly before giving the actual injection(s): "Normally when you feel a bit of discomfort, like the slight pinch from the injection, the tendency is to tighten up and hold your breath. But that doesn't really help you – it actually makes it feel worse. When your body stays relaxed and your breathing smooth, you feel much less discomfort. So, as soon as you feel the slight pinch, let that be a signal to you to intentionally relax and breathe through." As you give the injection(s), add: "That's right, nice and relaxed, breathing through, very good."

7.  During treatment, you may advise the patient: "Should you notice a bit of momentary discomfort, you immediately have a choice: focus attention on the discomfort, or return all of your attention to breathing/relaxation, gently breathing through the momentary discomfort. As you already know, focusing on discomfort tends to magnify it out of proportion. Like most patients, you will likely choose to remain focused on breathing/relaxation, allowing the discomfort to quickly fade away." Point out to the patient that he or she is in control of the situation. The patient continuously has the ability to return full attention to these techniques, thus minimizing any discomfort. If you notice the patient suddenly stiffen and hold his or her breath during a momentary discomfort, gently offer the reminder to breathe through and relax.

    Profound local anesthesia is of course a basic prerequisite. It should be understood that there is a tendency for anxious patients to misinterpret touch, vibration, smell, taste, and sound as "pain," giving the false impression that they're inadequately anesthetized.

8.  After the treatment is over, regardless of how the patient actually did, congratulate him or her for doing well. Encourage the patient, stating that the more this technique is practiced, the better he or she will be able to relax under other stressful conditions. With practice, the mind will be able to remain in this state of alert relaxation for longer and longer. With practice, muscular tension is greatly reduced, breathing remains deep and relaxed, and a greater sense of calm is enjoyed.

## Discussion

Mind–body therapies are increasingly popular. As the neurophysiologic mechanisms of therapies like meditation and hypnosis are elucidated, and their effects demonstrated and measured with advanced brain imaging techniques, these therapies are becoming increasingly accepted in mainstream health care (Jacobs, 2001).

The RR approach was preceded by a number of other well-known methods derived from modifying hypnosis and or meditation for clinical use. In the 1920s, Schultz modified hypnotic techniques to establish autogenic training (Schultz, 1959). In 1975, studying the effects of transcendental meditation (a form of concentration meditation) Benson suggested that all mind–body techniques (biofeedback, meditation, progressive muscle relaxation, tai chi, qi gong, yoga, etc.) elicit a common physiologic response he named the "relaxation response" (Benson, 1976). Since 1979, a great deal of clinical and research interest has been focused on Kabat-Zinn's "mindfulness-based stress reduction" (MBSR) program, based on mindfulness meditation and yoga (Germer, Siegel, & Fulton, 2005). All of these methods have scientifically proven effectiveness for a wide range of medical and psychiatric applications, but like the techniques upon which they're based, each requires significantly greater commitment in time and effort, by both clinician and patient, than is practical for most busy dental (or other) offices.

The primary goal of "mind–body therapies" is to produce sustainable positive behavioral changes. In contrast, the primary goal of RR is to keep the patient's attention anchored in the present, in order to prevent catastrophization right now, while being injected, and immediately afterwards, while being treated. Should the patient become motivated to practice meditation after experiencing the benefits of RR, long-term benefits would likely ensue, but this would be a secondary benefit.

Rapid Relaxation intentionally incorporates the positive suggestions of hypnosis. "Hypnosis happens when a subject is given some expectations for a change in awareness, the operator specifies the changes, and provides a cue for the change to happen"(Gibbons, 1979). But the change in awareness expected and specified by the operator guiding the patient to rest attention on the breath (concentration meditation) is in fact a state of relaxed alertness, the polar opposite of "dissociation of mind and body" typically associated with hypnosis. Traditional (formal) hypnotic inductions rely heavily on suggestions of "drowsiness" and "sleepiness", but an equally effective, less well-known form called "alert hypnosis" is compatible with mental alertness (Wark, 2006). Alert hypnosis is characterized by marked dominance of the sympathetic nervous system.

A subtle but important difference between RR and hypnosis relates specifically to the idea of trance. Hypnosis intentionally makes use of the human tendency to be in "trance," that is, to react according to set patterns, triggered by cues. Whether the cue is a signal taught by the hypnotherapist, or "buttons" we acquire through life events, there is a powerful tendency to react immediately, automatically, in a predictable fashion, be it useful (as per positive hypnotic suggestions) or harmful (overreacting to a minor event with rage). One of the most basic aims of meditation is to open up a time gap between a stimulus and one's response to the stimulus. This time gap permits conscious choice, precisely to override automatic responses, which are often inappropriate on reconsideration. Hypnosis and meditation both recognize that humans are usually in a state of trance. Hypnotherapists intentionally harness the trance phenomenon for positive therapeutic purposes, displacing harmful default trances. Meditation, as well as RR, aims at "waking up" from trances, so that one can respond appropriately to what is happening right now (instead of automatically based on a past event). Anxious patients are in a catastrophization trance, triggered by exposure to the dental environment. The RR approach, like concentration meditation, allows one to tolerate the experience so as "not to let affect come tumbling in" (Yassen, 2006). Both meditation and RR recognize how attention repeatedly drifts away from the focus of attention (feel of the breath). The skill learned in both is that of persistently, patiently, bringing attention back to the focus of attention. Attending to the ever-changing breath is literally linking attention to each successive present moment.

Hypnosis intentionally seeks to validate patients' expectations of achieving an "altered state" ("principle of trance ratification") (Hammond, 1990). The association of "a special state of mind" with formal hypnosis makes signing an informed consent advisable, and careful instructions, at the end of the session before leaving the office, to feel "refreshed and alert" mandatory. Since the principal focus of RR is awareness of what is happening in the present moment, its main "special" feature is that the patient is not in a trance, making informed consent and instructions to become alert unnecessary.

## In Summary

Rapid Relaxation is an extremely efficacious, simple-to-learn, straightforward method to help most patients undergo dental care with less emotional stress. Furthermore, using RR should not interfere in any way with the workflow of any dental practice where topical anesthetic is normally used. Most patients report positive experiences with RR. A large proportion of patients are clearly very pleased with it, whereas a very small proportion appears to simply ignore it. There does not appear to be any contraindication for use in patients who normally undergo dental treatment without sedative premedication.

# References

Baron, R.S., Logan, H., & Kao, C. F. (1990). Some variables affecting dentists' assessment of patients' distress. *Health Psychology*, 9, 143–153.

Benson, H. (1976). *The Relaxation Response*. Boston: GK Hall & Co.

Bub, B. (2006). *Communication Skills that Heal. A Practical Approach to a New Professionalism in Medicine*. Oxon, UK: Radcliffe Publishing Ltd.

Dionne, R. A., & Kaneko, Y. (2002). Overcoming pain and anxiety in dentistry. In R. A. Dionne, J. C. Phero, & D. E. Becker (Eds.), *Management of Pain and Anxiety in the Dental Office*. New York: WB Saunders Co.

Gavin, M., Litt, M., Khan, A., Onyiuke, H., & Kozol, R. (2006). A prospective, randomized trial of cognitive intervention for postoperative pain. *American Surgeon*, 72(5), 414–418.

Germer, C. K., Siegel, R. D., & Fulton, P. R. (Eds.) (2005). *Mindfulness and Psychotherapy*. New York: Guilford.

Gibbons, D. (1979). *Applied Hypnosis and Hyperempiria*. New York: Plenum Press.

Graham, G. (1998). Hypnosis. In P. Varley (Ed.), *Complementary Therapies in Dental Practice*. Oxford: Wright

Haase, O., Schwenk, W., Hermann, C., & Muller, J. M. (2005). Guided imagery and relaxation in conventional colorectal resections: A randomized, controlled, partially blinded trial. *Diseases of the Colon and Rectum*, 48, 1955–1963.

Hammond, D. C. (Ed.) (1990). *Handbook of Hypnotic Suggestions and Metaphors*. New York: WW Norton.

Hermes, D., Truebger, D., Hakim, S. G., & Sieg, P. (2005). Tape recorded hypnosis in oral and maxillofacial surgery – basics and first clinical experience. *Journal of Cranio-Maxillofacial Surgery*, 33, 123–129.

Hosey, M. T. (2002). Managing anxious children: The use of conscious sedation in paediatric dentistry. *International Journal of Paediatric Dentistry*, 12, 359–372.

Jacobs, G. D. (2001). The physiology of mind–body interactions: The stress response and the relaxation response. *Journal of Alternative and Complementary Medicine, 7*, (Suppl 1): S83–S92.

Kvale, G., Berggren, U., & Milgrom, P. (2004). Dental fear in adults: A meta-analysis of behavioral interventions. *Community Dentistry and Oral Epidemiology, 32*, 250–264.

Lundgren, J., Berggren, U., & Carlsson, S. G. (2001). Psychophysiological reactions in dental phobic patients during video stimulation. *European Journal of Oral Sciences*, 109, 172–177.

Meechan, J. G., Robb, N. D., & Seymour, R. A. (1998). *Pain and Anxiety Control for the Conscious Dental Patient*, (pp. 179–182). New York: Oxford University Press.

Milgrom, P. (2002). Nonpharmacologic methods for managing pain and anxiety. In R. A. Dionne, J. C. Phero, & D. E. Becker (Eds.) *Management of Pain and Anxiety in the Dental Office*. New York: WB Saunders Co.

Milgrom, P., Fiset, L., Melnick, S., & Weinstein, P. (1988). The prevalence and practice management consequences of dental fear in a major US city. *Journal of the American Dental Association*, 116, 641–647.

Moore, R., & Brodsgaard, I. (2001). Dentists' perceived stress and its relation to perceptions about anxious patients. *Community Dentistry and Oral Epidemiology, 29,* 73–80.

Olendzki, A. (2005). Glossary of terms in Buddhist psychology. In C. K. Germer, R. D. Siegel, P. R. Fulton (Eds.) *Mindfulness in Psychotherapy.* New York: Guilford.

Olendzki, A. (2006). *Meditation in Psychotherapy.* Continuing medical education course: Harvard Medical School (Spring, 2006).

Rausch, V. (1980). Cholecystectomy with self-hypnosis. *American Journal of Clinical Hypnosis, 22,* 124–129.

Schultz, J. (1959). *Autogenic Training. A Psychophysiologic Approach to Psychotherapy.* New York: Grune & Stratton.

Thompson, S. (1997). Hypnosis in the modification of dental anxiety. In M. Mehrstedt, & P. O. Wikstrom (Eds.) *Hypnosis in Dentistry.* Hypnosis International Monographs 3. Munich: M.E.G.-Stiftung.

U.S. Department of Health and Human Services (2004). *Advance Data From Vital and Health Statistics; No. 343 (5/27/04).* Hyattsville, MD: U.S. Government Printing Office.

Vassend, O. (1993). Anxiety, pain and discomfort associated with dental treatment. *Behaviour Research and Therapy, 31,* 659–666.

Wark, D. M. (2006). Alert hypnosis: A review and case report. *American Journal of Clinical Hypnosis, 48*(4), 291–300.

Yassen, J. (2006). *Meditation in Psychotherapy.* Continuing medical education course: Harvard Medical School (Spring, 2006).

## Chapter 7

# A Validation for Hypnosis in Dental Practice

*Gabor Filo*

## If Technology, Why Hypnosis?

Has the question intrigued you? Does it make you wonder about the implications? What is meant by technology and why would hypnosis even be considered in connection to it? Is hypnosis a superstitious vestige from the past?

In Dr. J. E. Dunlap's book *10 Trends: Dentistry's Emerging Directions*, written in 1986, numerous prognostications for the profession were remarkably astute and accurate. Many of the directions he outlined have indeed become the driving force of the profession. Among the 10 trends that have great significance today are: technological advancement, consumerism allied to holistic patient concerns, and to quote Dunlap directly "Dental Morale – from stressed to enthused."

Lasers, CAD-CAM fabrication, ever improving adhesives and porcelains, intra-oral cameras, and digital radiography are but a few examples of the technologies that have forever changed the nature of the profession. High touch is equated with high technology, but is it enough? Are these advances enough for a practice that is satisfying for all of the stakeholders – namely, the dentist, the staff and the patients? If one carefully looks at the other two referenced trends, then the answer to the question is a negative – they believe something more.

Melinda Davis, the CEO of The Next Group think tank, published her book *The New Culture of Desire: 5 Radical Strategies that will Change Your Business and Your Life* in 2002. It is the culmination of a six-year project by The Next Group, for big business clients addressing what humans want and what they do. They arrived at a startling conclusion: "Virtually every strategic excursion into the future has become an investigation into…the imaginational…what is known in some circles as non-ordinary or consciousness-based reality" (p. 9).

The Next Group concluded that in 1993, when governments relinquished control of the Internet, the world fundamentally changed. Humanity has started to live a virtual reality. In other words, for a greater part of the world, where daily subsistence is not an issue, our relationships to each other and the world changed dramatically. We "live" in our heads! However, this change has been subtle and concealed. Davis's work offers an in-depth explication of their observations and proffers five business models that are adaptable to the profession.

Technology is important for numerous valid reasons. However, it is no longer sufficient. An understanding of consciousness now is as important as being able to utilize an intra-oral camera. Understanding hypnosis aids in understanding consciousness issues. It offers solutions to some of these issues without having to get mired in the full spectrum of consciousness studies.

Before a working definition of hypnosis is addressed, a brief survey of our environment for covert and overt hypnotic techniques is illuminating. On any given day, any one of us may encounter these techniques: subliminal messages from marketers; Neurolinguistic Programming utilized by teachers or used car salesmen; Inner mental training®; visualization as adjunctive cancer care therapy or to enhance athletic performance; Super Learning®; Relaxation Response; autogenic training; meditation; EMDR for post-traumatic stress disorders. All of these techniques and modalities utilize the same innate fundamental characteristics of human consciousness.

Hypnosis has many faces and many definitions if it is to be the substrate for the above short list of modalities. Essentially, it is a social context-dependent set of psychophysiological processes that have a consensually accepted set of characteristics. To the dental practitioner, this does not convey an easily observable or usable meaning. Dr. Reginald Humphries, a psychologist, has promoted a definition that we witness daily in the course of interacting with people. He stated that: "Any marked dominance of either branch of the Autonomic Nervous System constitutes a trance." Hypnosis is a subset of a continuum of altered states of consciousness referred to as "trances."

An aside: As in all areas pertaining to hypnosis, trances, and altered states of consciousness, taxonomy is debated. There is at present no generally agreed upon definition of hypnosis or for that matter any altered state of consciousness. Thus, to use the term "trance" may be considered archaic, but for our purposes it merely suggests that the Western model of hypnosis as it is commonly understood is a subset of other similar entities.

Generally, we experience four classes of trance. Relational trances occur when one person is deeply absorbed in another. Hopefully, we have all experienced this trance. Situational trances are deep absorption in an activity. Csikszentmihalyi (1993) called this *flow*. Root canal therapy on $MB_2$ of an upper second molar would qualify. Inner-mind trances are hypnotic, meditative, and daydreaming for example. These may be individually or heterogeneously induced, with or without mechanical or chemical aids. Lastly, group mind trances are those in which an individual is the carrier of the values, mores, and characteristics of a particular group. If the group is large in number, then it is a cultural trance. The globe is ablaze with the extreme demonstrations of this phenomenon.

One of the quintessential features of trances is the ease by which they can be reactivated or re-induced once they have been initially experienced. This, perhaps, is the most salient point of our discussion. Once a trance has been experienced, it can become like a continuous loop videotape. Press the right button, and it plays forever. Sadly, the replaying of a "tape" happens so quickly and subconsciously that it is usually too late to alter it. Hence, our interpersonal issues erupt. A great deal of energy and conscious focus is required to go through the day without letting our buttons be pushed. All of us have examples from our daily lives – spouses, children, certain patients, and even non-human occurrences that engender a fixed and constant response. Pavlov would indeed be proud. This can, and usually does, lead to stress or more specifically distress, but more on this later.

A dental example of this recurring trance is dentally anxious and phobic patients. They usually have acquired their phobia as children. Every time they are exposed virtually or *in vivo* to dentistry, their video loop plays, maintaining their fear and reinforcing it. As adults they know cognitively that their fears are irrational, but the loop, that is, the trance, is overriding their cognitive understandings.

Hypnosis in dentistry has both physiological and psychological uses. A brief inventory of dental applications includes the following. Hypnosis may be used to reduce the quantity of chemical anesthetics (local and general), analgesics, and sedatives. It complements nitrous oxide use and may be used as a substitute anxiolytic or supplement for surgical anxiety premedication. The psychological and physiological components of gagging may both be controlled hypnotically.

Acute and chronic pain management is possible, as is the enhancement of denture adaptation. Hemorrhage and salivary flow may be regulated as required. Habit management, from digit sucking to bruxing, has been supported with hypnotic interventions. Patient management and motivation may also be enhanced with hypnotic techniques.

Let us briefly examine the factors mitigated by hypnotic techniques from the perspective of each of the participants in a dental interaction. Patients have the ability to modulate their psychological and physiological responses. They can also manage their anxiety levels, acute and/or chronic pain, and any maladaptive habits. Time distortion is available to them. Personal growth through goal achievement is also feasible once self-hypnosis is mastered.

Staff members, akin to the patients, may also manage their personal stress and utilize hypnotic techniques for personal goal achievement. Understanding hypnotic principles enhances patient management and interpersonal communications. There is an inherently timesaving benefit when interpersonal interactions are made easier.

Clinicians may also garner these same benefits. Underlying all of the foregoing advantages is the common thread of stress (distress) and its management. An easy-to-read work on the insidious nature of chronic stress is *When the Body Says No,* which is by Gabor Maté (2004).

This is the second profound conclusion that The Next Group discovered in their work. Not only are we living in our heads as it were, but the digital age that we have created has also detrimentally increased our stress levels. To quote: "An inescapable stream of technoaccelerated mind traffic collides with an increasingly battered human psyche" (p. 56). Thus, for all of us, any transaction now becomes a state-of-mind cost/benefit analysis. Be honest, what would you really like to do to the person who invented voicemail?

So, what does this mean? If one is knowledgeable about hypnosis, hypnotic techniques, and the trances we live, then one is in a position to enhance one's well-being. This then accrues benefits not only in the office, but also in one's personal evolution. To acquire the benefits, you do not ever have to become a practicing hypnodontist, but certainly understanding this "soft" technology enhances one's personal and professional life.

## *The Acquisition of Hypnosis*

How does one go about acquiring the requisite skills to employ hypnosis in practice? One could certainly read about it and experiment, but a formal training program would be more efficient. In Canada there are several professional organizations that have as their primary mission to instruct professionals and then offer a continuing forum after the initial training. Most of the provinces have a clinical hypnosis association, and the umbrella organization is the Canadian Federation of Clinical Hypnosis. They may be found at www.clinicalhypnosis.ca. In the United States, the counterpart is the American Society of Clinical Hypnosis, which can be contacted at www.asch.net. Both organizations offer various workshops and training sessions throughout the year.

Once trained, not unlike the alchemist of old, the refinement process is a lifelong adventure. When working with patients, the general principle has been to present oneself as believable and sincere. Thus, we never use scripts. Hammond's magnum opus, *Handbook of Hypnotic Suggestions and Metaphors* (1990) contains many fine scripts and suggestions for all manner of patient problems. The recommendation is to be familiar with the general format of the script, know the lynchpin phrases and then make it one's own. Rote memorization is to be avoided; rather an understanding of the material is the goal so that one can adapt it to the patient as the session circumstances vary. This approach permits a degree of freedom for the operator and allows the requisite creativity that a hypnotic session engenders.

# Integrating Hypnosis into Dental Practice

Once the decision to use hypnosis is in place and one has acquired the requisite knowledge and skills, the question becomes: how is hypnosis actually integrated into practice?

The question can best be answered from two different perspectives – that of practice management and that of the clinical applications.

## Practice Management Perspectives

On the second day of the second year of this author's dental education, in a course referred to as patient management, the comment was made that hypnosis works, but you can't run a practice that way. This perspective was often repeated by other colleagues at the time. That may have been true with the then-current state of knowledge about hypnotic techniques, but perhaps it merely reflected a lack of information or an unwillingness to explore other paradigms of practice.

Just as styles of hypnosis may be characterized as authoritarian and permissive, the integration of it may be said to be either formal or informal. Before elaborating on this further, several more characterizations of hypnosis will be addressed.

Clinicians may be said to be authoritarian, paternalistic, directive or permissive, maternal, or non-directive in the style of hypnosis that they employ with a patient. Each style has its optimal use. Similarly, hypnotic states or trances may be passive, passive-alert, or active-alert in nature. Further, to employ Dr. Humphries's definition and schema, one can speak of sympathetic or parasympathetic trances exhibiting beneficial attributes to pathological attributes.

So, let us examine the formal trance or hypnotic session in a dental practice. The underlying assumption for this discussion is a fee-for-service private practice office setting. It may be a single practitioner operation or a multipractitioner facility with many auxiliaries.

The patient has presented for hypnosis for some dental-related issue. This individual may have been referred, found the practice by way of some component of the practice marketing, or the clinician may have suggested it as an appropriate modality. If the patient is new to the practice, a formal intake process is required. This would include the usual collection of demographic information and a comprehensive medical and dental history. As in regular dental care, one would never work on a stranger. Hypnotic interventions are no different.

If the patient is one of record, then the intake process is abbreviated to only those issues pertaining specifically to the use of hypnosis. In this instance, however, specific questioning about psychiatric care and psychological issues is also appropriate. Consultations with the patient's general practitioner or psychiatrist/psychologist may be necessary before hypnotic interventions commence. A patient's psychiatric history is not a contraindication for the use of hypnosis by dentists, but the hypnosis must be utilized knowledgeably and carefully.

Patients are accustomed to filling out health-related forms in medical and dental practices. A hypnosis-specific form to elicit information about the patient's interest in hypnosis is useful. This also validates in the patient's eyes that although this is unique care, it also fits into the usual dental milieu.

Having patients write out their answers as a patient "statement" before working with them is informative. It permits one to screen for problems outside of one's capabilities and experience, or jurisdictionally determined scope of practice. Patients' compliance is also revealed by the degree to which they offer information. An opportunity to actively participate in their own care is offered, which is unusual in the medical/dental model most patients know. This also forms the basis of the "therapeutic contract" between clinician and patient.

Minimally, the questions should include:

- How did you come to know about our office?
- What do you know about hypnosis?
- Have you ever been hypnotized before and for what?
- What was the outcome of that experience?
- What do you wish hypnosis for at the present time?
- How do you think hypnosis will help you in this instance?
- How will this change your life?

- Since all hypnosis is self-hypnosis, are you willing to actively participate in your treatment?

Answers to these queries should permit one to determine if the patient's expectations are realistic. The last question helps screen out the patient who has a problem, but wishes to give it to the clinician. We all have denture stories in which we have become just another statistic in a long line of incompetents.

The preceding questions also begin the process of informed consent. Each one offers a springboard to addressing the myths and misconceptions about hypnosis.

As we know, allaying the fears of a patient should foster cooperation and compliance, and minimize resistance. Rapport is created and enhanced.

Hypnotic treatment plan formulation is also expedited by answers to the foregoing questions. Skilful interviewing should generate enough information to facilitate inductions for whichever style and trance type is appropriate for the patient.

As described, this formal intake process could take up to an hour or more. Consultations may be in order before the hypnotic treatment plan may be completely formulated. An additional appointment may be made with the patient to discuss the treatment plan and the time it will require.

Clinicians may like to break up the hypnotic interventions into several appointments that may or may not be coupled with dental care. All of these have a consequence to the practice flow – the scheduling of appointments. It also has an overhead and profitability consequence that must be borne by the patient.

Private practice dental economics, at least in North America, tend to be predicated on leveraging time – that of the doctor, hygienists, assistants, and administrative staff. Some of the intake process can be delegated to auxiliaries to mitigate impact on scheduling. In a multioperatory practice, this is easier than in a one or two operatory facility. Ultimately, the clinician will have to be involved and the clinician time is more costly than auxiliary time

Each formal hypnosis session will involve at least three people – the patient, the doctor, and an auxiliary in the capacity of chaperone regardless of the patient's gender. Those used to seeing the business side of dentistry not just the therapeutic aspects will immediately appreciate the full overhead ramifications. Thus, formal hypnosis sessions in a dental practice will be overhead weighted and the cost to the patient will have to be appropriate to permit this type of treatment intervention. Private practice settings will vary from institutional dental practices, which by their nature may be able to offset the costs to the patients.

Individual dental procedures have different time requirements and differing profitability. Many procedures are loss leaders, so it may be with formal hypnosis. However, for the loss up front with formal hypnosis, the return will be at the back end with the fee-for-service dentistry that its use facilitates.

Informal hypnosis is the complement to the formal session. It does not have any of the trappings of the formal session. The patient has had a formal intake into the practice for exclusively dental needs and concerns. That is to say, that the clinician has familiarity with the patient. It is predicated on recognizing the patient's physiological state – sympathetic or parasympathetic dominant – and intervening accordingly.

Ericksonian, or permissive styles of hypnosis, are the foundation for this type of intervention. Many times all that is required is a method by which local anesthetics may be administered in a comfortable manner. Usually, the intervention consists of the particular patter of the clinician that forms the therapeutic communication that facilitates the injection.

Appropriate communication, that is hypnotic language and the utilization of hypnotic techniques, is all that is required to enhance the desired outcome of the dentistry. There is no extra overhead associated with this type of hypnotic intervention. It is done on the fly, so to say.

This does, however, bring to light another potential concern. In the formal utilization of hypnosis, a process takes place that is the foundation of informed consent. Informally applied techniques, albeit beneficent in intention, lack this process. Ethical issues may arise by utilizing these techniques for the practitioner. Each of us has to determine whether or not our actions could engender an ethical breach and act accordingly.

## Clinical Applications

A review of the dental applications of hypnosis is laid out in the following text box. Note that there are two broad areas, psychological and physiological applications. Neither category is purely one or the other. There is substantial overlap between the two categories. Nor is this listing exhaustive. Imagination and creativity are the only true limitation to the possible applications.

# Dental Applications

### Psychological

- dental fear, anxiety, and phobia

- reduction in chemical anesthetics, analgesics, and sedation – complement to $N_2O$

- supplement or substitute for surgical premedication

- gagging: control of excessive "reflex"

- habit management

- motivation: oral hygiene

- patient management

### Physiological

- bruxing control

- pain management: acute and chronic

- denture adaptation

- control of hemorrhage and salivary flow

- treatment of syncope

General dental practitioners will note that most dental procedures hold the potential to be enhanced with hypnosis. As with any treatment modality, careful patient selection is a must.

Another perspective on the clinical integration of hypnosis is that of what hypnotized people do and what they experience. The following categorizes the types of phenomena that the hypnotized patient may "do." Each phenomenon also lists the dental application for its evocation, but it also illuminates what the patient may be experiencing. The experiential component can only be known for certain by asking the patient. Here too, each phenomenon may have multiple applications and may represent many different internal experiences for the patient.

| Phenomena | | Dental Application |
|---|---|---|
| Ideomotor phenomena: | → | induction methods and training control of patient physiology |
| – hands moving together | | |
| – arm lowering | | |
| – eye closure | | |
| – ideomotor signals | | |
| – passive arm catalepsy | | |
| – levitation | | |
| – inhibition of voluntary control | → | trance ratification, trance deepening |
| – automatic movements | | |
| – finger lock | | |
| – eye catalepsy | | |
| – limb rigidity/immobilization | | |
| Ideosensory activities | → | trance ratification |
| Dissociation | → | "safety" mechanism – "safe room" |
| Analgesia & anesthesia | → | minimize or replace local/general anesthetic |
| Hypnotic dreams | → | appointment rehearsal reframing previous issues |
| Post-hypnotic suggestion | → | treatment suggestions behavior modification, re-induction cue |
| Hyperamnesia & age regression (partial and revivification) | → | reframing a past experience |
| Amnesia | → | amnesia for dental experience or a component |
| Time distortion | → | change perception of treatment duration |
| The hidden observer or ego-state phenomena | → | bruxing/habit awareness |
| Hallucinations – negative & positive – visual, auditory, kinesthetic, olfactory, gustatory | → | modification of treatment experience, e.g., impressions |
| "Classic suggestion effect" – experiencing phenomena | → | trance ratification, deepening with sense of involuntariness |

# Dental Applications

## Dental fear, anxiety, and phobia

Studies of dental avoidance suggestive that from 5 to 40% of the population who do not seek dental care at least once annually do so out of fear. Sadly, an afternoon spent with an inquisitor has greater appeal to these folks than a visit with the dentist. Even excrutiating dental pain may not be sufficient to drive these people into a dental office to get acute care.

Regrettably, most dental curricula devote minimal time to psychology in general – the psychology of the mouth only in passing. Thus, before a discussion about hypnosis as an intervention for anxiety is approached, basic definitions should be addressed.

Fear, anxiety, and phobia tend to be utilized interchangeably. Clinically, working with the patients, this may not matter. To better understand the dynamics of the patient's experience and to better tailor an intervention for that particular individual, a clear understanding of the concepts is crucial. The following definitions should demonstrate the relationships between these concepts.

### Fear
- the general term for the anxiety and agitation felt in the presence of danger

- an individual's emotional response to a perceived threat or danger

- physiologic changes modulated primarily by sympathetic nervous system, i.e., tachycardia, profuse perspiration, hyperventilation, muscle tension, GI upset, emotional arousal

- overt behavioral movements, i.e., jitteriness, shakes, pacing, attempts to escape, or avoid the perceived threat (Milgrom et al., 1995)

### Anxiety
- responses to situations in which the threat is ill-defined, ambiguous, or not immediately present (Milgrom et al., 1995)

### Phobia
- marked and persistent fear of clearly discernable circumscribed objects or situations (American Psychiatric Association, 1994)

- stimulus provokes an immediate anxiety response

- stimulus avoidance is of such proportion that it causes significant distress or interferes with one's social or role functioning (Milgrom et al., 1995)

Perhaps it may not be obvious from the definitions, but there is a progression from the state of fear to phobia. Essentially, it is a conditioned response. Over time, the fear may become an ingrained phobia where the distress of anxiety is the facilitating emotional and physiological factor.

Other terms that are used clinically and in the literature are descriptions of the genetic and temporal nature of anxiety. These concepts are self-explanatory.

*Trait anxiety*
- a characteristic range of anxiety responses that is relatively fixed is a personality trait

*State anxiety*
- an anxiety response in a particular time and situation

*Acute anxiety*
- high and maladaptive acute anxiety; over time, beyond the stimulus, it can develop into chronic anxiety (Maxmen & Ward, 1995)

*Chronic anxiety*
- uniformly high and maladaptive trait anxiety

If one studies the literature about dental anxiety and phobia, many definitions, patient classifications, and concepts abound. Sadly, as is the case with most specialties and subspecialties, the professionals may be talking about the same thing, but are incapable of understanding each other. As someone once said about the common English language separating the British and Americans, so it is with researchers from the different backgrounds. The following is an example of terminology that exists, but is not well known or used outside the dental arena.

*Exogenous anxiety*
- psychological in nature involving situational anticipatory anxiety symptoms

*Endogenous anxiety*
- a disease that does not respond to rest, relaxation, and behavior modification exhibiting a more severe cluster of symptoms from within

## Natural History of Endogenous Anxiety

Stage I       Subpanic symptom attacks
Stage II      Polysymptomatic panic attacks
Stage III     Hypochondriasis
Stage IV      Limited phobic avoidance
Stage V       Social phobias
Stage VI      Extensive phobic avoidance (agoraphobia)
Stage VII     Secondary depression

(Rubin et al., 1988)

In North America the most commonly used set of psychiatric descriptions is the Diagnostics and Statistics Manual version IV. The manual correlates its diagnostic categories with the International Classification of Diseases (ICD-10). The numbers preceding the DSM-IV descriptions are the ICD codings. Anxiety disorders are listed below. As can be seen, they cover a wide range of disorders, both psychological and systemic in nature.

## DSM IV Anxiety Disorders (APA, 1994)

300.01     Panic Disorder without Agoraphobia

300.21     Panic Disorder with Agoraphobia

300.22     Agoraphobia without history of Panic Disorder

300.29     Specific Phobia (formerly Simple Phobia) → dental phobia is listed under this

300.23     Social Phobia (Social Anxiety Disorder)

300.3      Obsessive-Compulsive Disorder

309.81     Post Traumatic Stress Disorder

308.3      Acute Stress Disorder

300.02     Generalized Anxiety Disorder (includes Overanxious Disorder of Childhood)

293.89          Anxiety Disorder due to…[indicate general medical condition]
  –  cardiopulmonary disorders
  –  temporal lobe epilepsy
  –  pheochromacytoma
  –  hypoglycemia
  –  hyperthyroidism
  –  post-concussion syndrome
  –  delerium
  –  alcoholic anxiolytic withdrawal
  –  caffeine overuse
  –  other stimulants and other drugs

300.00          Anxiety Disorder not otherwise specified

Dentally anxious patients may not have only one anxiety disorder – specific or simple phobia – but may have several. Needles, injections, and the drill are the usual provoking stimuli for specific phobias. However, other issues may also have an impact on the patient's behavior. This is vital information for the clinician when working with this population of patients. Interventions for specific phobias are less complicated than for more complex phobia disorders. Dentists who work with these patients should be regularly consulting with the patient's mental health care professional. Should the patient not have one, it is incumbent upon the dental clinician to suggest a referral when a more complex problem is suspected.

In traditional anxiety and phobia treatment interventions, the object is ultimately to change the patient's physiological, cognitive, and affective response to the dental setting and experience.

Physiologically, some form of parasympathetic nervous system (PSNS) tone-enhancing exercise is taught. In an anxiety-provoking situation, the sympathetic nervous system – the flight or fight response – is overreacting. Since both halves of the Autonomic Nervous System cannot be overreacting concurrently, the PSNS tone is enhanced. Progressive muscle relaxation is the usual method taught to these patients.

To address the cognitive and affective components of the phobia, the patient is exposed either virtually or *in vivo* to his or her fears. Coping skills for both the cognitive and affective components are taught in order to face these fear-provoking stimuli. In the following table, the usual psychological treatment types are listed for Specific or Simple phobias. Included in the table is the number of sessions required on average for progress. Also referenced is the addition of hypnosis to the treatment to enhance these procedures.

A computer metaphor may illuminate the value of hypnosis in treating anxiety and phobia patients. Consider the mind as using DOS for its operatons. The phobia has become a subroutine in some part of the programming, essentially a recursion formula. Most people need help to manipulate the commands in DOS to accomplish their goals. It's not user friendly. So, for the great majority of us, Windows is the interface between the machine and DOS that lets us actually do the things we wish to accomplish. It facilitates accessing the machine, just as hypnosis does with any of the therapies customarily employed for treating anxiety disorders.

## Treatment of Specific Phobias with Behavior Therapies and their Hypnotic Enhancements

| Treatment modality | Sessions | Time per session | Hypnotic enhancement |
|---|---|---|---|
| Imaginal Flooding | 5–10 | 45'–60' | – *trance utilized for relaxation and dissociation*<br><br>– *flooding of past traumatic experience* |
| **Graduated exposure** (Extinction)<br><br>– *in vivo*<br>– in imagination<br>– videotape | 6–10 | 30'–60' | – *in hypnosis* in vivo *exposure or imaginally as required*<br><br>– *TV; blackboard; video screen; theatre techniques to expose to anxiety inducing scenes*<br><br>– *"control" dials for phasing out stressful scenes and replacing with scenes where patient exhibits coping skills* |
| Systematic desensitization with muscle relaxation | 10–15 | 30' | – *in trance, patient exposed to hierarchy of fears*<br><br>– *double dissociation technique for extremely phobic*<br><br>– *self-hypnosis practice recommended with customized audiotape*<br><br>– *future pacing* |
| **Modeling** – mastery and coping<br><br>– *in vivo* or symbolically (videotape) | As required | As required | – *in trance state to expedite process* |

| Treatment modality | Sessions | Time per session | Hypnotic enhancement |
|---|---|---|---|
| Stress Inoculation<br><br>i) Phase I – instruction in pain/fear and subjective role<br><br>ii) Phase II – selecting/devising set of coping skills, e.g.:<br>– distraction<br>– cognitive transformations<br>– self talk<br><br>iii) Phase III<br>– integrating into active coping plan by practicing under fire | 6 | 30′ | *– in trance, patient is asked to imagine stressful situation focusing on usual thoughts, physiologic responses, beliefs and freezing these*<br><br>*– patient is asked to modify each of these modalities with positive responses and to observe the new responses*<br><br>*– purpose is to give the patient control and to alter negative thought patterns* |
| Self-administered Stress Inoculation (do-it-yourself manual) | 15 | 5 days/ 3 weeks | *– self-hypnosis would facilitate and possibly shorten time required* |
| Psychodynamic techniques<br><br>– uncovering procedures<br>– age regression<br>– affect bridge<br>– dream inductions<br>– time projection | | | *– all can be utilized with hypnosis to enhance the technique or shorten the time commitment* |

Synthesized from: Rubin, Kaplan, & Kaplan (1988), The dental clinics of North America, *Dental Phobia and Anxiety*, 32(4), and Mehrstedt & Wikstrom (1997) *Hypnosis in Dentistry*.

This overview of hypnosis and dental anxiety is very brief. In-depth information may be found in the references. The seminal work by Milgrom et al. (1995), *Treating Fearful Dental Patients: A Patient Management Handbook*, 2nd edn, is the starting point for a grounding in dental anxiety. Wester and Smith's (1991) *Clinical Hypnosis: A Multidisciplinary Approach* offers excellent information on the utilization of hypnosis.

In sum, a quote from Kay Thompson (Kane & Olness, 2004) is appropriate: "Hypnosis offers one method for making dentistry more tolerable for the frightened patient. The patient can be taught to go into the trance state with the understanding that he will then be able to handle the dental situation with comfort, dignity and control."

# Suggested Reading

## General

Hambleton, R. (2002). *Practising Safe Hypnosis: A Risk Management Guide.* Carmarthen, Wales: Crown House Publishing.

Lynn, S. J., & Rhue, J. W. (Eds.) (1991). *Theories of Hypnosis: Current Models and Perspectives.* New York: Guilford.

Rhue, J. W., & Lynn, S. J. (Eds.) (1997) *Handbook of Clinical Hypnosis.* Washington, DC: American Psychological Association.

Simpkins, C. A., & Simpkins, A. M. (1991). *Principles of Self Hypnosis: Pathways to the Unconscious.* New York: Irvington.

Wester, W. C., & Smith, A. H. (1991). *Clinical Hypnosis: A Multidisciplinary Approach.* Cincinnati, OH: Behavioral Science Center.

Wier, D. R. (1996). *TRANCE: From Magic to Technology.* Ann Arbor, MI: Trans Media, Inc.

## Historical Dental References – Hypnosis and Psychosomatics

Fross, G. H. (1966). *Handbook of Hypnotic Techniques with Special Reference to Dentistry.* Irvington, NJ: Power Publishers, Inc.

Frost, T. W. (1959). *Hypnosis in General Dental Practice.* Chicago, IL: The Year Book Publishers, Inc.

Landa, J. S. (1953). *The Dynamics of Psychosomatic Dentistry.* Brooklyn, NY: Dental Items of Interest Publishing Company, Inc.

McDonald, A. E. (1949). *Psychosomatics and Hypnotism in Dentistry.* New Orleans: published by author.

Mehrstedt, M., Mehrstedt, P., & Wilksröm, O. (Eds.) (1997). *Hypnosis in Dentistry.* Stiftung, Germany: Hypnosis International Monographs, M.E.G.

Moss, A. A. (1953). *Hypnodontics or Hypnotism in Dentistry.* Brooklyn, NY: Dental Items of Interest Publishing Company, Inc.

Ryan, E. J. (1946). *Psychobiologic Foundations in Dentistry.* Springfield, IL: Charles C. Thomas Publisher.

Shaw, S. I. (1958). *Clinical Applications of Hypnosis in Dentistry.* Philadelphia, PA: W.B. Saunders.

Simpson, R., Goepferd, S., Ogensen, R., & Zach, G. (1985). *Hypnosis in Dentistry: A Handbook for Clinical Use.* Springfield, IL: Charles C. Thomas.

Stolzenberg, J. (1950). *Psychosomatics and Suggestion Therapy in Dentistry.* New York: Philosophical Library, Inc.

## Dental References for Psychology

Croucher, R., & Kent, G. (1998). *Achieving Oral Health: The Social Context of Dental Care* (3rd edn). Oxford: Wright.

Eli, I. (1992). *Oral Psychophysiology: Stress, Pain and Behavior in Dental Care*. Boca Raton, FL: CRC Press, Inc.

Feinmann, C. (Ed.) (1999). *The Mouth, the Face, and the Mind*. Oxford: Oxford University Press.

Horowitz, L. G. (1986). *Overcoming Your Fear of the Dentist*. Rockport, MA: Tetrahedron, Inc.

Jagger, R., & Enoch, D. (1994). *Psychiatric Disorders in Dental Practice*. Oxford: Wright.

Kroeger, R. F. (1987). *Managing the Apprehensive Dental Patient*. Cincinnati, OH: Heritage Communications.

Weiner, A. A. (1994). *The Difficult Patient: A Guide to Understanding and Managing Dental Anxiety* (2nd edn). Randolph, MA: Review Publishing Co.

# References

American Psychiatric Association (1994). *Diagnostic and Statistical Manual of Mental Disorders DSM-IV* (4th edn). American Psychiatric Association.

Csikszentmihalyi, M. (1993). *The Evolving Self*. New York: Harper Collins.

Crabtree, A. (1997). *Trance Zero: Breaking the Spell of Conformity*. Toronto: Somerville House Publishing.

Davis, M. (2002). *The New Culture of Desire: 5 Radical Strategies that will Change Your Business and Your Life*. New York: The Free Press.

Dunlap, J. E. (1986). *10 Trends: Dentistry's Emerging Directions*. Tulsa, OK: PennWell Publishing Co.

Eli, I. (1992). *Oral Psychophysiology: Stress, Pain and Behavior in Dental Care*. Boca Raton, FL: CRC Press, Inc.

Fricker, J., & Butler, J. (2000). *Natural Health®: Secrets of Hypnosis*. New York: DK Publishing.

Hammond, D. C. (1990). *Handbook of Hypnotic Suggestions and Metaphors*. New York: W.W. Norton.

Kane, S., & Olness, K. (Eds). (2004). *The Art of Therapeutic Communication: The Collected Works of Kay F. Thompson*. Carmarthen, Wales: Crown House Publishing.

Maté, G. (2004). *When the Body Says No: The Hidden Cost of Stress*. Toronto: Vintage Canada.

Maxmen, J. S., & Ward, N. G. (1995). *Essential Psychopathology and its Treatment* (2nd edn, revised for DSM-IV). New York: W.W. Norton.

Mehrstedt, M., & Wilkstrom, P. O. (Eds.) (1997). *Hypnosis in Dentistry*. Stiftung, Germany: Hypnosis International Monographs, M.E.G.

Milgrom, P., Weinstein, P., & Getz, T. (1995). *Treating Fearful Dental Patients: A Patient Management Handbook* (2nd edn). Washington, DC: Continuing Dental Education University of Washington.

Rubin, J., Kaplan, G., & Kaplan, A. (Eds.) (1988). The dental clinics of North America. *Dental Phobia and Anxiety*, 32 (4).

Schlitz, M., et al. (Eds.) (2005). *Consciousness & Healing*. St. Louis, MO: Elsevier.

Wester, W. C., & Smith, A. H. (1991). *Clinical Hypnosis: A Multidisciplinary Approach*. Cincinnati, OH: Behavioral Science Center Publications.

## Chapter 8

# Pain, Anxiety, and Dental Gagging in Adults and Children

*Ashley A. Goodman and Donald C. Brown*

Hypnosis is an altered state of awareness in which individuals withdraw their peripheral awareness and concentrate on a focal goal. It is the process of communication with an individual directly toward an unconscious response to suggestion. It is not sleep. It is a deep state of concentration rather than relaxation. Communication is maintained and is direct to the subconscious. Suggestion is the process of accepting a proposition for belief in the absence of intervening and critical thought that would normally occur. The absence of critical thought distinguishes suggestion from persuasion. The indication and manipulation of expectations are vital components. A placebo is a form of suggestion but a suggestion is not a placebo.

## History

The following is a brief revision of the history of hypnosis and the major figures in it. Grouping of suggestions to achieve a trance began in Egypt: Ebers papyrus (1000 BC); "temple sleep." "Druidic sleep," Druids. Mesmer magnetic fluid theory "Animal Magnetism" was discredited in 1784. John Elliotson (1791–1868), Professor of Theology and practitioner of medicine at London University and past president of the Royal Medical Society, performed painless surgery in the 1840s. He promoted the use of the stethoscope (Crasilneck & Hall, 1985).

James Braid replaced the "Animal Magnetism" theory with the concept of suggestion; anesthesia by suggestion. In 1847 he discovered that all the major effects of his newly termed "hypnosis" could be induced without sleep. Braid was considered the "Father of Modern Hypnosis."

Hippolyte Bernheim wrote books about hypnosis and psychological conditions. Later in his career he used formal hypnosis less and less. He found that the same results could be obtained by suggestion in waking state. Hypnosis was at the peak of general acceptance from 1860–1900, but that period was followed by a rapid decline in acceptance and use in surgery with the introduction of chemical anesthetics (nitrous oxide). Freud used hypnosis initially but later discarded it in favor of psychoanalysis.

In 1955, the British Medical Association endorsed hypnosis for certain purposes. It was recommended that all physicians and medical students receive training in hypnosis (*British Medical Journal*, April 23, 1955). Three years later, an editorial in the *Canadian Medical Association Journal* (1958) recognized the therapeutic benefits of hypnosis and urged acceptance of the British Medical Association's report.

In the same year as the Canadian Medical Association's action, the Council on Mental Health of the American Medical Association (AMA) was moved to endorse hypnosis, that is, the council's report endorsed the therapeutic use of hypnosis by medical and dental professionals.

In 1958, the American Medical Association accepted hypnosis in medical practice as a therapy. In 1965, the Canadian Medical Association accepted hypnosis in medical practice and medical school curricula. In 1961, the American Psychiatric Association accepted hypnosis as a specialized psychiatric procedure.

In 1960, two years after the AMA's approval, the American Psychological Association endorsed hypnosis as a branch of psychology (Hilgard, 1965, p. 4). Subsequently, the Council on Mental Health of the AMA (1962) recommended 144 hours of hypnosis training over a 9- to 12-month period at undergraduate and postgraduate levels of medical training. Ultimately, hypnosis had been given a professional stamp of approval (Scheflin & Shapiro, 1989).

# The Nature of Trance

## Trance

Every patient's trance is a bit different. One can't always tell if one is in a trance because it may only take the form of a change in perceived environment or an increase in receptivity to suggestion. In a response to the complex set of suggestions that make up a hypnotic induction, the patient experiences a narrowing of attention and pays less attention to their external environment and more to the actual process. The person listens more intensely to the therapist and if the suggestions don't conflict with his or her moral views and values, he or she will comply. Many patients who demonstrate a hypnotic appearance do not respond to *suggestions*; others' response appearance can be changed by appropriate suggestions without affecting the response to suggestions. It may sometimes be distinguished externally by a sleep-like appearance with a fixed and glassy stare, psychomotor retardation, etc. and internally by a calm dissociated state with possible perceptual distortion and amnesia. The ability to remember and retain control always remains with the patient.

## Variations of Susceptibility

In general, the best hypnotic subjects have been found to be curious, adventuresome, and imaginative; more hypnotizable than a competitive, controlled, and/ or fearful individual. The rough breakdown is as follows: 5% non-suggestive; 95% light trance; 55% medium trance; 20% deep trance. Children are susceptible to hypnosis and more susceptible than adults. They reach a susceptibility apex at about age 9. Between the ages of 6 and 9 there is a steady gain in susceptibility. After age 9 there is a gradual decline until about age 15 through the early 20s, then a leveling off with normal adult susceptibility. Individuals are more susceptible to hypnosis in mid-childhood than at any other time in their life. Approximately, 80–90% of the population can be hypnotized to a useful level for pain or anxiety control. If left alone for 10–20 minutes, a deeply hypnotized patient may come out of a hypnotic trance unassisted.

Voluntary muscles can be induced into deep relaxation or rigidity. Involuntary muscle tone can be influenced and effects on heart rate, blood pressure, bleeding, and salivation are demonstrable. All five senses can be influenced. Visualization, concentration, and memory can be greatly enhanced. With the introduction of nitrous oxide, patients can hear suggestions but their memory of the suggestions is temporarily blocked. Patients are significantly more responsible to suggestions for behavior change after removal from nitrous oxide than those who have not had nitrous oxide.

## Levels of Hypnosis

The following list offers brief definitions of levels of hypnosis.

### Waking suggestion
Controversial level recognition. Increased suggestion receptiveness.

### Hypnoidal
Lightest trance response with extreme relaxation. Eyes closed, sometimes eyelids fluttering. Similar to pleasant drowsiness prior to natural sleep. Traditional rapport is established.

*Light trance*
Breathing slower and deeper with slower muscle activity. Posthypnotic suggestibility. Suggestions will be potent and effective. Tense anxious patients become relaxed. Eyes closed.

*Medium trance*
All of the above. Varying degrees of analgesia (glove anesthesia). Partial amnesia and some catalepsy (muscular rigidity). Some control of fainting, bleeding, saliva flow, gagging.

*Deep trance (Somnambulism)*
Patients can open their eyes without awakening. Amnesia without suggestion. Surgical anesthesia and positive and negative hallucinations can be demonstrated. Patients may appear alert and awake. Eyes may be open. Speech normal and muscle activity is not impeded.

*Posthypnotic Suggestion*
A suggestion given during hypnosis to take effect after the trance state has terminated.

*Autohypnosis*
Related to the ability of the patient to enter hypnosis, when he or she wants to, independent of the presence of the therapist

# Dental Applications of Hypnosis

The following outlines basic applications of hypnosis for dentistry.

Behavior control – the professional has the responsibility for behavior management, including relaxation and anxiety control. Hypnosis can be used for fear elimination, i.e., future expectations are built upon past experiences; perceptual confusion (apples vs. oranges); time distortion. It may also be used for quelling undesirable habits, such as tongue thrust, reverse swallowing, TMJ dysfunction, bruxism, clenching. Amnesia – Children are better than adults (73–80%) with hypnosis. Analgesia, anesthesia, pain control. Prevention of gagging and nausea. Control of saliva and bleeding. Restorative appliance tolerance, pretreatment desensitization. To improve self-image, self-esteem, and confidence.

Hypnotic Techniques – Some things to keep in mind: secure the patient's attention. Entry into a child's world must be at their level, and allowance should be made for a shorter attention span with more fantasy and imagination. For adults and children, similar communication representational modes should be utilized.

Interview – The interview should encompass the following components: patient history, desensitization, preinduction and induction, explain myths and misconceptions of hypnosis. Techniques used include: informal induction, waking suggestion, and semantics. Constant monologue with proper word choice. Voice control – softer, quieter. Body language – smooth, gentle, slow movements. Metronomic cadence to carotid pulse – tympanic membrane artery. Creative visualization – involve multiple senses for best results.

Reframing – symptom substitution. Change in perspective. Secondary benefit assessment. NLP (Neurolinguistic Programming) – breathing and set-up of trigger point for relaxation. Distraction and sensory confusion – needleless syringes, taste of anesthetic vs. ice cream, rewards (toys), glove balloons. Concurrent use of nitrous oxide. Nitrous oxide produces an altered state of consciousness similar to hypnosis. Facilitates and deepens normal and resistant patient induction.

## Stages of induction

The following outlines the typical stages of induction. Preinduction or mindset is used to develop a state of positive expectancy in the patient, leading to rapport and acceptance of the trance state. An explanation of hypnosis is provided as an opportunity to alleviate any patient concerns. This is a good time for indirect suggestions. The patient should relax, concentrate, and give free run to his or her imagination. The patient voluntarily agrees to let the mind and body behave involuntarily, and be responsive to suggestions of the therapist.

The essential conditions for effective use are motivation, removal of doubts and fears, and fixation of attention. When attention is fixed, the field of consciousness becomes narrowed and the unconscious mind becomes accessible. Suggestions then slip past the conscious mind and enter the subconscious where they are accepted without criticism. Relaxation prevents anxiety arousal. The limitation of voluntary movements, monotony, and suppression of all ideas except those upon which attention is to be concentrated are important. Most failures to induce hypnosis are due to a lack of adequate preinduction of the patient and the patient's perception of a lack of confidence on the part of the therapist.

- *Tests for susceptibility* – ability to accept suggestions in the waking state are optional. Such tests are brief.

- *For the induction of trance* – sensory intake is at a minimum while the patient's motor activity is held at a minimum. Repeated suggestions are given in a monotone voice for relaxation, heaviness, and sleep. The therapist should look for physiological changes in the patient, such as eye movement, facial and body muscle relaxation, and deeper, slower breathing.

- *For deepening or stepping the trance* – a reinforcement of the induction stage to produce greater patient relaxation and compliance to achieve a thera-peutic level is facilitated. The "Spiral of Belief" is established, meaning the patient has experienced certain things happening after their occurrence was predicted by the therapist. The therapist reminds and allows further time for the processes in the situation to deepen: "Breathing will relax you more; background noises only serve to help focus your concentration, visualiza-tion is better and takes you deeper into a more pleasant, relaxing feeling." There is a continual focusing on internal stimuli and mental imagery.

- *In the utilization or suggestion phase* – hypnotic and posthypnotic therapeutic suggestions are given. The suggestions are for desired behavior along with cues to incite the desired response. All suggestions made within hearing distance of the patient should be positive. Staff members should be alerted. "Ego strengthening" suggestions and reinduction triggers are presented. Posthypnotic suggestions for "autohypnosis" with memory, reinforcement, and trance strengthening are made. Any continuing unwanted suggestions regarding a changed state (numb hand, etc.) *must be removed*.

- *In the rising and signal to awaken phase* – the level of patient relaxation and hypnosis are lightened and the expectation suggestion for awakening is introduced. Once out of arousal with the signal given, and after reinforcing suggestions, allowance for a return to wakefulness must be made including giving adequate time to arouse comfortably. A rising tone incorporates sug-gestions for feeling refreshed, wide awake, and a pleasure to be associated with the hypnotic experience.

## Formal Induction

The formal induction includes the following features. There is obvious guiding of the patient with recognizable steps. Eye fixation and progressive relaxation are integral components. Suggestions of eye fatigue and heaviness culminate in eye closure and further suggestions deepen the trance. Suggestions are made to bring relaxation to sections of the patient's body. Eye fixation, progressive relaxation, and distraction are primarily for patients who try to analyze. In another approach, the patient counts backwards from a high number.

- *The raised arm levitation* – have the patient visualize one hand with weights and then the other with helium filled balloon(s) or ball in bucket, sand-filled bucket, etc. Guided imagery: A TV show or movie is projected on closed eyelids and it becomes clearer as relaxation proceeds. This works well with children. Rapid inductions: Eyes open wide, look up at top of head; let eyelids relax and close and relaxation spread to the rest of body.

## Informal Induction

An informal induction can be distinguished in the following ways. In indirect hypnosis, communication can be verbal and nonverbal (body language, touch, story-telling). Subliminal use of hypnotic suggestion bypasses most of the anxieties that cause resistance and reduces the time needed. Time is one of the main reasons that the use of hypnosis took a back seat to pharmacological sedation in behavioral modification and anesthesia/analgesia.

Behaviors that are traditionally associated with hypnosis can occur without "formal" hypnotic induction. Induction is not a monotonous, repetitive monologue by the therapist. The induction does not cause hypnotic behavior, but merely defines the situation, for instance, role-playing may be necessary.

Permissive suggestions, rather than authoritarian, are featured. Patient's responses are utilized, i.e., when eye closure is not readily forthcoming, then the therapist discontinues those suggestions and continues with drowsiness and tiredness, which may lead to eye closure; or how relaxing keeping the eyes open might be. The emphasis is on the patient's and their hypnotized intrapsychic functioning (subconscious). Indirect, paradoxical, and permissive suggestions cause the patient to act in certain hypnotic ways. Patients will experience and qualify their hypnotic modified behavior if the therapist communicates in such a way that the patient/clients have little alternative but to respond hypnotically. Suggestions are often sophisticated, subtle, and given in a roundabout way (as in metaphor).

Obscure and integrated therapy, which is not obvious to the patient, requires informed consent. This is not time-consuming. Suggestions can be spoken to the nurse, with the patient present, and still be effective: "You may notice how relaxed and comfortable he/she appears while sitting in a dental chair. His/her enjoyment and pleasure will increase with time and the number of visits." Appearance is more "mystic" than in formal trance approaches when the suggestions are acted upon.

In Neurolinguistic Programming (NLP), behavior for every given person is patterned and predetermined. How individuals interact with their world, and how they can change their interpretation of this world to alleviate their distress and/or induce behavior modification to assist coping with their life more effectively, is already set. The primary representational system for communication is already there: Visual (I see what you mean); Auditory (I hear what you're saying); Kinesthetic (I feel that I understand you); Olfactory (I smell a rat); Gustatory (It leaves a bad taste in my mouth). The first three options are the more common ones.

The direction of gaze provides many clues: upward accessing visual information; horizontally accessing auditory information (left–recall; right–constructing); downward to left accessing auditory information; downward to right is kinesthetic; gaze not focused in distance is visual. Communication with the patient is verbally in his or her representational system (involving all five senses) and also at an unconscious level by tone, phrase emphasis (analogue marking), and movement. Anchors (triggers) for the patient's conditioned response are in the patient's communication mode. Pitfalls of hypnosis include headaches, confusion, anxiety, and drowsiness. Other issues might include delayed effects of posthypnotic or uncancelled hypnotic suggestion, or misunderstanding of suggestions. Abreaction – spontaneous emotional outpouring due to the surfacing of repressed memories – might result. Although this is central to certain types of therapy, it may occur inadvertently during a normal induction in which sympathetic support and encouragement to go naturally through the abreaction must be given. Transference and countertransference are defined as strong positive or negative patient feelings toward the therapist by identification with someone from the past. Countertransference is an emotional involvement of the therapist with the patient.

Restriction of use of hypnosis to the therapist's field of expertise is very important.

Patients with a history suggesting psychiatric disorders of endogenous depression should be treated by an experienced therapist in the field. A careful history taking is important.

*In Closing*
No recipe has been given for hypnotic induction. This is because the technique must vary according to the professional, patient, situation, and objective. However, learning subliminal behavior modification can greatly enhance patient management and stress reduction.

# Dental Fear, Phobias, and Pain in Adults

Nearly one half of the people in the United States express some fear toward dentistry. This fear ranges from mild apprehension to paralyzing anxieties. Approximately 30 million of these individuals have a fear so great that they are termed phobic and avoid dental care completely. Numerous edentulous patients never have dentures made or have dentures they never wear because of overt gag responses (Zach, 1990).

Gerschman, Reade and Burrows (1980) present an excellent chapter on "Hypnosis in Dentistry" covering historical development, psychology of the orofacial region, indications, anxiety and fear, the production of dental analgesics, the control of syncope, anaesthesia and sedation techniques, the control of gagging, salivation and bleeding, postoperative pain and discomfort, and the disadvantages and limitations of hypnosis.

In 1843, John Elliotson, a distinguished British physician well known for his introduction of the microscope to Great Britain, published a book entitled *Numerous Cases of Surgical Operations Without Pain in the Mesmeric State*. He described in detail his personal use of the mesmeric state for the treatment of chorea and rheumatism. He also presented the work of his colleagues, who were able to perform such procedures as the painless release of contractures, incision of abscesses, and dental extraction. A contemporary of Elliotson's, James Braid, introduced the term *hypnosis* derived from the Greek *hypnos* (sleep). Braid was credited with the elucidation of the psychological aspect of hypnosis and the power the mind has over the body. Spiegel and Bloom state that hypnosis has been found to be an effective analgesic since the nineteenth century and reported their randomized clinical trial on group hypnosis therapy to reduce metastatic breast carcinoma pain in 1983.

Manusov (1990) presents two cases to demonstrate clinical applications of hypnotherapy. Hypnosis has been a therapeutic tool for centuries. The Egyptians used "sleep temples" in which therapeutic suggestions were made, and kings were often thought to have healing powers. The clinical applications, however, have not been elucidated until recently.

In Manusov's first case, hypnosis is used to alleviate pain in a gravid patient in sickle cell crisis. In the second case, a 27-year-old woman presented to the family practice clinic because of a severe dental phobia. As a child she had sustained an avulsion of the maxillary incisors, which required multiple surgical procedures. Over the previous five years, she had been unable to obtain either routine dental care or daily dental hygiene because of fear and an exaggerated oral sensitivity. Hypnotherapy was offered as a treatment option, and a combination of desensitization and suggestion was used to alleviate her fear. After a comfortable level of trance was obtained, she was told to imagine how great the feeling was as she walked out of a dentist office. In trance, after she was able to imagine herself having completed a dental examination, she was progressively led through the dental examination, beginning from calling for an appointment through to the actual procedure. Ultimately after several months of hypnotherapy, she was able to care for her teeth and undergo dental examination. The desensitization, by slowly obtaining cognitive control over fears, resulted in the resolution of her phobia. The historical, theoretical, and clinical applications were reviewed.

Hermes, Truebger, Hakim and Seig (2004) reported that during a one-year-trial period, 209 operations under combined local anesthesia/medical hypnosis were carried out on 174 non-preselected patients between the ages of 18 and 87 years old. The surgical range covered oral, plastic and reconstructive, onco-logical, septic, and trauma operations. Medical hypnosis treatment conditions for both patient and surgeons were achieved in 93% of cases. The conclusion is that controlled clinical studies are not necessary to obtain objective data on the effectiveness of hypnosis-induced intraoperative effects in oral and maxillo-facial surgery. It can be concluded that a rational, widely accepted method, free of side-effects to improve surgical conditions, is currently not in use. Hypnosis is such an option. It has been used in various surgical fields and dentistry for at least 50 years. Positive intraoperative effects of hypnosis include sedation, anxiolysis, inhibited motor skills, and increased tolerance towards physically and psychologically demanding surgical procedures. Overall preparation time (information, seedings, and induction) is approximately 15 minutes, with com-plete postoperative reorientation of the patient within less than 1 minute. The technical costs associated with hypnosis when compared with established phar-macological procedures must be counted as yet another advantage.

Moore, Brodsgaard and Abrahamsen (2002) report a three-year study of dental anxiety treatment outcomes: hypnosis, group therapy, and individual sensi-tizations vs. no specialist treatment. All of the therapeutic interventions were effective in dental anxiety reduction and improved trust at the end of the spe-cialist training period and after test dental treatments on a population of odonto-phobics with known and previously described characteristics.

Outcomes of hypnotherapy, group therapy, and individual systematic desen-sitization on extreme dental anxiety in adults aged 19–65 years old were com-pared by regular attendance behaviors, changes in dental anxiety, and changes in beliefs about dentists and treatment after three years. Treatment groups were comparable with a static reference control group of 65 anxious patients (Dental Anxiety Scale > 15) who were followed for a mean of nearly six years. After three years, 54.5% of hypnotherapy patients, 69.6% of group therapy, and 65.5% of systematic desensitization patients were maintaining regular dental care habits. This was better than the 46.1% of the reference group, who reported going regularly to the dentist again within the cohort follow-up period, and 38.9% of a control subgroup with observation for three years. Women were bet-ter regular attenders than men at three years. Specialist-treated regular attend-ers were significantly less anxious and had more positive beliefs than regular attenders from reference groups.

The results were robust even though they favored the whole group, which was observed for a longer period and thus had greater opportunity to establish regular care habits than did intervention groups. All specialist-intervention, three-year regular attenders were also significantly less anxious and had more positive beliefs about dentists than regular attenders from the whole control group. Regression model results confirmed that regular attenders receiving specialist treatment had reduced their dental anxiety more effectively at three year follow-up than had three year subgroup control attenders. It could be concluded from the present data that many anxious patients can successfully start and maintain regular dental treatment on their own, despite years of treatment avoidance owing to negative dental beliefs and related phobic or extreme anxiety.

The "balance of power" within the dentist–patient relationship requires that busy, often stressed dental practitioners note and address the anxiety or pain perceptions of patients or that patients become more assertive about their needs. Dentists must provide patients with a sense of trust that they will take the time to explain procedures, provide reassurance, obtain adequate anesthesia from the patient's perspective, and encourage patient participation in their own treatment. Thus, in general, it must be concluded that the process of trust in dentist–patient relations should be promoted as a primary therapeutic goal that enables patients to improve beliefs about dentists and dentistry while also confronting and controlling their anxiety and avoidance of dental care. The present results also indicated that in order to achieve long-term regular dental care attendance after specialist treatment it is also important for specialists to provide adequate counseling that would benefit regular dental-care habits. Patients should be helped to learn to attribute their success mainly to their own efforts and not the therapist's, so that they may successfully continue regular dental health care in private practices of their choice after initial therapy.

Elkins, Jensen, and Patterson (2007) reviewed 13 controlled prospective clinical trials of hypnosis for the treatment of chronic pain. Their findings indicate that hypnosis interventions consistently produce significant decreases in pain associated with a variety of chronic pain problems. Most of the hypnosis interventions from chronic pain include instructions in self-hypnosis.

The hypnosis intervention group demonstrated an overall decrease in pain ($p < .0001$) for all sessions combined. The mean rating of the effectiveness of self-hypnosis practice outside the sessions was 6.5 on a 0–10 scale. Their current revision indicated that hypnotic interventions for chronic pain results in significant reductions in perceived pain that in some cases may be maintained for several months.

Thompson (1994) describes a case where hypnosis was used to facilitate anxiety management and to alter the negative "catastrophic" cognitions of a very anxious, medically compromised man. Treatment was carried out using hypnosis in combination with inhalation sedation; the successful outcome was construed as a positive experience so that the pattern of dental avoidance was finally broken. Mr. K tolerated procedures presented in a calm, graded, sympathetic manner with hypnosis and adjunctive use of nitrous oxide and local anesthetics, and as he coped with the received treatment, this acted as a positive reinforcement which helped to provide the motivation and incentive to come for subsequent treatment.

Hammond (1990a) presents a "Suggestions in Dental Hypnosis" (pp. 183–196) section covering most of the common problems in one's practice.

Alladin, Sabatini and Amundson explain lucidly the criteria for "Evidence-Based Practice in Clinical Hypnosis" (2007). On the same issue, Hammond (2007) provides an updated review of the literature on the effectiveness of hypnosis in the treatment of headaches and migraines, concluding that it meets the clinical psychology research criteria for being a well-established and efficacious treatment and is virtually free of the side-effects, risks of adverse reactions, and ongoing expense associated with medication treatments.

Néron and Stephenson (2007) report a systematic and critical review of the evidence on the effectiveness of hypnotherapy for emesis, analgesia, and anxiolysis in acute pain. Clinical hypnosis in cancer settings provides symptom reduction (pain and anxiety) and empowers patients to take an active role in their treatments and procedures.

Kvale, Berggren, and Milgrom (2004) did a meta-analysis of behavioral interventions in adults with dental fear. The aim of their meta-analytic and systematic quantitative approach was to examine the effects of behavioral interventions for dental anxiety and dental phobia. Eighty studies were identified where dental fear treatment with behavioral methods was evaluated – 38 of 80 met entry criteria and were included in a meta-analysis. Some 3 to 5% of the adult population in Western societies suffers from dental phobia, while up to 40% of the adult population have been reported to be fearful of dental treatment. It seems reasonable to infer that the heterogeneity primarily refers to some underlying differences in sampling that do not seriously reduce the validity of the reported changes.

Several of the controlled studies performed on patients with severe dental anxiety seeking care at a specialized clinic found the condition treatable and the change lasting. Montgomery, David et al. (2002), report a meta-analysis on the effectiveness of adjunctive hypnosis with surgical patients. The goal of their study was to estimate the effectiveness of adjunctive hypnosis in controlling signs and symptoms after surgery. The meta-analysis revealed a significant benefit of hypnosis with surgical patients. The overall beneficial effect of hypnosis with surgical patients was significant.

In this sample of studies, 14 of the hypnosis interventions included live administration by a health care professional, and eight of the interventions relied solely on audiotapes. Effect sizes for both randomized and non-randomized studies were significantly more than zero (P < 0.05), indicating that both types of study design revealed impressive benefits because of hypnosis. The present meta-analysis revealed that on average 89% of surgical patients in previous studies benefited from adjunctive hypnosis interventions relative to patients in control conditions.

Both self-report and objectively assessed end points were influenced. This suggests that, in a general sense, adjunctive hypnosis is a powerful tool for addressing signs and symptoms after surgery. That is, adjunctive hypnosis helped the majority of patients reduce adverse consequences of surgical interventions. We found no evidence to support the position that these findings were dependent on the method of the hypnosis administration or study design.

Some 89% of surgical patients in hypnosis groups benefited relative to control patients. These data are consistent with previously published meta-analyses on hypnotic analgesia generally, as well as socio-cognitive views of hypnosis and experimental studies. All suggest that hypnosis can be used to alter patients' expectations for their own benefit. It has been posited that randomized clinical trials underestimate the effects of psychological interventions.

The present results provide strong support of the efficacy of hypnosis with surgical patients, but the question of the mechanism by which it functions remains to be determined. There must also be a physiological substrate for any psychological mechanism, and recent studies have found physiological correlates of hypnosis with brain-imaging techniques (e.g., positron emission tomography and electroencephalograph techniques). (Montgomery, David et al., 2002).

Gerschman, Reed, and Burrows (1980) report that the role of hypnosis in the relief of pain has further been elaborated by the results of the clinic. It is clear from the types of pain successfully treated that hypnosis is able to reduce or eliminate both "sensory" and "suffering" pain. Pain problems ranging from those of predominately psychogenic origin to those of predominately organic origin can be managed.

Hypnosis does not merely produce relaxation and relief from anxiety and thus make pain more tolerable, it is capable of reducing pain itself, sometimes completely, sometimes reducing it to acceptable levels. This evidence is clear from both experiences with laboratory subjects and with patients in pain presenting to the orofacial pain clinic.

The most recent meta-analysis on hypnosis in chronic pain by Elkins, Jensen, and Patterson (2007) demonstrates that the findings indicate that hypnosis interventions consistently produce significant decreases in pain associated with a variety of chronic pain problems.

The hypnosis intervention group demonstrated an overall decrease in pain ($p < .0001$) for all sessions combined. The mean rating of the effectiveness of self-hypnosis practice outside the sessions was 6.5 on a 0–10 scale.

## Summary

Information about stimulus transmitted to CNS by peripheral fibers is now available. Spinal cord or fifth nerve nucleus signals are facilitated or inhibited by other peripheral nerve fiber signals. Descending control systems that originate in the brain modulate the receptiveness from the transmitting cells.

It is thought that the higher cortical centers are inhibited during deep hypnosis, preventing pain impulses from coming into awareness. Pain is a signal that something is amiss, whether physical or psychogenic. Diagnosis should be made before attempting treatment. Chronic pain may also appear as a conversion symptom and present atypically. "I live with the pain" may be interpreted by the subject subconsciously as "If I didn't have the pain, I'd be dead."

Hypnosis doesn't remove the pain (objective findings are the same), but it merely reduces the perception of it. The pain is registered, but it is ignored. Pain can't just be "commanded" away.

Psychological variables can exacerbate or reduce the subject's appreciation of the physical "pain" stimulus. Pain responses are not only of a physical nature (somatogenic origin), but also are attenuated by many psychological variables such as anxiety, focus of attention, expectations, the subject's interpretation of what the "pain" is, secondary gain, conversion symptom, and various psychopathologies, etc. Excellent rapport and trust is needed between patient and therapist. The patient requires high motivation. Organic and psychogenic pain can be experienced in differing ratios. For psychological pain, the origin or underlying problem must be attended to first. It must be determined that there is no organic problem or secondary benefit (attention, avoiding work, gaining sympathy, worker's compensation payments, circumventing responsibilities, etc.).

## Anxiety

When the fear of pain is reduced, the perception of it becomes more tolerable. Pain threshold varies greatly from individual to individual. The greater the fear, anxiety, and anticipation, the lower is the threshold for that individual. In addition, relaxation may relieve muscle pressure on nerves.

A complete history is essential and should encompass as complete a description of the pain as possible, including the patient's imagery of pain (color, dull, stabbing, etc.). The same description, with appropriate attenuation, should be used when giving suggestions for "creative visualization" for "healing," meaning: "A picture is worth a thousand words" in treatment. Using the subject's representational mode of communication, when possible, is effective: visual, auditory, kinesthetic, olfactory, and gustatory.

Anatomical interpretation is not exact, but rather is the patient's interpretation; therefore, the exact area should be explained and delineated. "Glove anesthesia" may be interpreted by patient as being only superficial.

The chief disadvantage of hypnosis is the unpredictability of the level of effectiveness. Some pain may be alleviated with the first session. For most, relief will be attained after a few sessions. Some subjects might notice immediate relief, whereas others find relief delayed for several hours. As with other uses of hypnosis, the same degree of results with every subject, or with the same subject every time, cannot be assured. At best 10–15% of patients find hypnosis to be effective for surgery and over the long term. For another 30–40% of patients, hypnosis is used for minor surgery etc. in moderate depth.

Once the cause of the subject's pain is diagnosed and found to now be non-useful, it is *important not to eliminate all pain*, but to selectively attenuate only that non-useful pain, and advise the subject accordingly. It may be best to leave some "sensation" so that patient won't exacerbate the problem. A time limit may be necessary with decreasing numbness, but retained analgesia if a prolonged effect is desired; otherwise analgesia should be removed prior to re-alerting.

With regard to induction/suggestions, authoritarian/direct suggestions work best with rapid induction and stroking of the affected area for acute pain. Permissive/non-authoritarian suggestions with normal induction are appropriate for reducing the anxiety accompanying the pain experience in less emergent situations.

A combination of hypnosis and anesthetics/analgesics (medium trance) generally results in fewer anesthetics and/or analgesics being necessary. There is less effect on cough or gag reflex. Placebo effect is present 50% of time. The combination is good for poorer surgical risk patients, including debilitated, geriatric, and so forth. Posthypnotic suggestions, autohypnosis, ego-strengthening, glove anesthesia, etc. allow for fewer opiates to be effective, thus reducing negative side-effects. Antidepressant medication may be necessary if pain has been present for an extended time.

There is disassociation of the individual from his or her pain, and the patient becomes an observer (moderate–deep) of the pain (Hilgard & Hilgard, 1975). Age regression or progression (not in terminal patients) should be made to a time when pain was not present, or will not be present and thus how comfortable that time is will be quite effective. Subjective awareness is reduced in the patient.

## Perceptual Distortion

This approach allows pain to be substituted to a level that is tolerable and/or more comfortable, e.g., a more comfortable numbness. There is displacement to a more easily controlled part of body, for example, transference to the hand and subsequent evaporation. Progressive diminution of pain can be encouraged through switches, volume control, and the like. Sometimes a suggestion for an increase in the pain may be necessary prior to analgesia/anesthesia so that the subject can make a comparison of the changed sensitivity. This also demonstrates that they can control the pain.

## Expanding Relief by Distraction

In this sense, distraction means focusing on those areas of the body that feel comfortable and visualizing those areas of comfort expanding and relieving the uncomfortable areas and diluting the discomfort. This method combines well with "progressive relaxation." With extreme pain, sometimes the best focal point is the pain itself, which then can be varied in intensity as in the following.

Use creative visualization to form a mental image of the pain. Then incorporate deep, regular breathing with the imaging. The pain is diminished and blown out with each exhalation, and fresh healing air is brought in, along with an alteration of the visualized image of the pain (diminution in size, or fading of colors, etc.).

"Autogenic training" is a desensitization technique whereby the treatment procedure is previewed verbally while the patient is under hypnosis. The result may include faster healing, with less pain postsurgery, less chemo-analgesia/ anesthesia required, and fewer airway problems.

Hypnosis for pain control is better reinforced when done in the morning. The subject has time to "program" for greatest duration of comfort with more anticipated distractions. Practice with self-hypnosis multiple times during the day also allows for the greatest reinforcement.

Patients can be reassured by being told by the health care professional that he or she believes in their pain, its intensity, and will provide support. Ego-strengthening suggestions should be provided. Patients should be guided to understand that they can control the level of the "pain" and that their control will increase with practice and understanding. The process should be explained to improve expectancy and "role playing" can be used to bolster confidence.

The sessions and suggestions for posthypnotic self-hypnosis can be recorded to allow the subject "practice time" for self-analgesia, multiple reinforcement, etc.

## Pain, Anxiety and Hypnotherapy with Children

Hypnotherapy has been used with children for more than 200 years. Olness and Kohen (1996) note that pediatric dental patients respond to a variety of hypnotic techniques to achieve pain control. Numerous cases are delineated by them in detail with many references (pp. 276–281). The authors speculate that this was a function of excellent local anesthesia which left little pain to reduce. Gokli, Wood et al. (1994) explain that behavior management is critical to the success of pediatric dental procedures. They found that children tended to become involved in novel and intriguing imaginative situations, and that their attention was diverted from the painful medical procedure. This suggests that children's attention can be held and sustained through the use of imagination and fantasy. The technique of hypnosis alters the state of consciousness by narrowing the patient's field of attention to one idea through intense imaginative involvement.

Spiegel and Peterson (1980) found that preschool children taught such coping skills as relaxation, pleasant imagery, and calming self-talk, all similar to hypnosis, demonstrated significantly less distress in the dental office setting than a non-taught control group. In another study, children receiving instruction in relaxation and positive self-talk (i.e., calming thoughts, positive reappraisals, and self-reinforcement) exhibited fewer stress-related behaviors during dental procedures than children in control and non-treatment groups.

Twenty-nine children between the ages of 4 and 13 years old participated in the study. The hypnotic procedure was accomplished in the operatory by instructing the patients to take deep breaths through the nose, to relax, and to concentrate on their favorite visual imagery or sensations.

Statistically significant differences in pulse rate attributable to the hypnosis condition were noted. Pulse rate decreased at the time of injection in hypnotized subjects by 4 bpm, whereas it increased at this point in non-hypnotized patients by 10 bpm. This is attributable to the hypnotized patients' relaxed state, their attention being successfully held, even during the physical stimulation of injection. In summary, hypnosis can have a positive impact on pediatric patients for injection of a local anesthetic.

Biobehavioral strategies that encourage children's participation in treatment, thereby mobilizing coping and recovery skills, are increasingly being recognized as a necessary and potent part of pediatric clinical practice.

Children under the age of 6 years old shift very easily from one cognitive state to another. It is these blurred boundaries between reality and fantasy that allow the young child to rapidly enter an altered state of consciousness in which sensations, perceptions, and experience can be changed (Kuttner, 1991).

Nearly half the people in the United States experience fear of dental treatment, from apprehension to paralyzing anxiety. Objectives in the use of hypnosis are to reduce anxiety, fear, discomfort, and distress, and to improve cooperation, self-control, self-mastery, and expectations for the future. Children from 3 to 5 years of age experience blurred boundaries between reality and fantasy that allow them to enter an altered state of consciousness rapidly (Rustvold, 1994).

Anxiety and fear are significant determinants of both attendance patterns and behavior during dental treatment. Fear-motivated dental avoidance in these studies ranged from 8% to 16%, which is considerably higher than the often quoted estimates of 5–6% of some 20 years ago (Gerschman, 1989).

In a randomized controlled study of 52 children, Lambert (1996) evaluated the effects of hypnosis/guided imagery on the postoperative course in children. The research questions were: (1) What are the effects with guided imagery versus routine preoperative nursing preparation on the child's length of hospital stay, preoperative pain medication requirements, and pain rating? (2) What is the effect of hypnosis with guided imagery versus routine preparation on the child's state of anxiety? Each child's average pain score was used for comparison between the groups. Lambert found that the average length of hospital stay was significantly shorter for the experimental group, 5.0 days compared with 5.8 days for the control group ($p < 0.5$). The children in the experimental group rated their pain significantly lower (mean 3.9) than the children in the control group (mean 4.4) ($p < 0.1$).

Butler, Symons, Henderson, Shortliffe, and Spiegel (2005) report a study that was designed to examine whether relaxation and analgesia facilitated with hypnosis could reduce distress and procedure time for children who underwent voiding cystourethrography exams (VCUG). Forty-four children were randomized to receive hypnosis (n = 21) or routine care (n + 23) while undergoing the x-ray procedure. Those who were randomized to the hypnosis condition were given a one-hour training session in self-hypnotic visual imagery by a trained therapist. Parents and children were instructed to practice using the imaginative self-hypnosis procedure several times a day in preparation for the upcoming procedure. The therapist was also present during the procedure to conduct similar exercises with the child.

Outcomes included child reports of distress during the procedure, parents' reports of how traumatic the present VCUG was compared with the previous one, observer ratings of distress during the procedure, medical staff reports of the difficulty of the procedure overall, and total procedural time. The present findings are noteworthy in that this study was a controlled, randomized trial conducted in a naturalistic medical setting. In this context we achieved a convergence of subjective and objective outcomes with moderate to large effect sizes, including those that may have an impact on patient care and procedure costs that were consistently supportive of the beneficial effects of hypnosis – a noninvasive intervention with minimal risk. The findings, therefore, have immediate implications for pediatric care.

Milling and Constantino (2000) in a review of controlled studies on the efficacy of clinical hypnosis with children revealed promising findings, particularly for reduction of acute pain, chemotherapy-related distress, and injuries.

Montgomery, DuHamel and Redd (2000) in a meta-analysis of 18 studies revealed a moderate to large hypnoanalgesic effect, supporting the efficacy of hypnotic techniques for pain management. The results also indicate that hypnotic suggestion was equally effective in reducing both clinical and experimental pain. The overall results suggest broader application of hypnoanalgesic techniques with pain patients.

Peretz and Bimstein (2000) in a study of the use of imagery suggestions during administration of local anesthetic in children found that the pulse rates of hypnotized children decreased and the observed levels of crying were lower. In addition, hypnosis was more successful among younger children. Moreover, it was found that susceptibility to suggestions, first measured between 5 and 6 years of age, increased until ages 12 to 14 years old and gradually decreased as age increased. Facial expression, eye movement, and body tonus were found to be reliable behavioral measures. This study demonstrates that most of the children could conjure up images or accept suggestions during the process of dental injection.

General anesthesia is still commonly used in the United Kingdom for extractions in anxious children unable to accept local anesthetic (Shaw & Welbury, 1996). An alternative is inhalation sedation, where a controlled mixture of nitrous oxide and oxygen inhaled through a small nasal mask is used to sedate the child. This technique has been shown to be safe and effective in children for restorative treatment and minor oral surgery procedures. Hypnosis has been shown to be effective in reducing anxiety in children receiving dental treatment. Preliminary reports suggest there may be a beneficial effect from hypnosis when used in conjunction with inhalation sedation. One hundred and seventy-nine children were seen in the sedation and extraction clinic. In 34 cases it was necessary to stop treatment. From this group of children those who could at least accept a dental examination were considered for hypnosis. Children were selected if eye closure was attained. A five-minute informal hypnotic induction was used to relax the child and focus his or her awareness inwardly. Once accepted, the imagery was developed for an additional ten minutes using the senses with which the child found it most comfortable to work. Each approach was tailored to the individual, the clinician leading the imagery through simple questioning and suggestion. The treatment and hypnotic imagery were continued simultaneously until placement of the gauze pack to achieve homeostasis. The child was then praised and the posthypnotic suggestion given that the warm "comfy" feelings would remain upon opening his or her eyes (Shaw & Welbury, 1996).

Additional information may be found in the following books: *Behaviour Management in Dentistry for Children* by G. Z. Wright (1975); *Handbook of Hypnosis and Psychosomatic Medicine* in the contribution from Gurschman, Read, and Burrows (1980); *A Child in Pain: How to Help, What to Do*, by Leora Kuttner (1996); *Handbook of Hypnotic Suggestions and Metaphors* in the contribution from D. Corydon Hammond (1990); and *Trance and Treatment: Clinical Uses of Hypnosis* by Spiegel and Spiegel (2004).

## *Summary*

The following is an outline of parameters, choice points, and options when working with children.

### *Introduction*
Children don't respond well to intellectual abstractions, and exhibit more unpredictable behavior. Pain control in children involves the use of anesthetics, and the reduction of anxiety. A misinterpretation of pain with anxiety is common.

*Anxiety Precursors*
In the category of "uncontrolled" we put: Previous untoward experiences – dental or medical. Peer preconditioning. Parental preconditioning. Miscellaneous – general media exposure.

In the category of "controlled" we put: Fear of the unknown. Office ambiance – children's books, pictures, peaceful atmosphere. Staff/doctor attitude. Parental attitude and support – parents accompanying children. Establishment of rapport and trust. Miscellaneous – short "child oriented" initial appointments.

*Situational Priorities*
Acute emergency – scared versus spoiled, show-off, long-term treatment.

*Current Practice*
Physical restraint by staff: Hand-over-mouth, towel technique, papoose boards, pedi-wraps, mouth props. Sedation: Better circulation – medications take effect faster and more profoundly, but are of shorter duration. Dosage reliant.

During general anesthesia, lower body weight results in greater chance for toxicity etc.

*Tell! Show! Do!*
Dialoguing at child's level and positive reinforcement with friendliness are used during the introductory visit to seed positive future experiences.

*Adolescent Hypnosis*
Behavior control – the professional has the responsibility for behavior management, relaxation, and fear elimination. It must be remembered that future expectations are built upon past experiences. Options include perceptual confusion (apples vs. oranges), quelling undesirable habits, and amnesia. Children do better than adults (73–80%) with hypnosis, analgesia, prevention of gagging and nausea, control of saliva and bleeding.

# Background

Children are more susceptible to hypnosis than adults, reaching a susceptibility apex at about 9 years old. Between the ages of 6 and 9 there is a steady gain in susceptibility; after age 9, there is a gradual decline until about age 15 through the early twenties, and then leveling off with normal adult susceptibility.

Individuals are more susceptible to hypnosis in mid-childhood than at any other time. "A child's wakeful state seems less removed from the hypnotic state than an adult's. Older individuals seem to counteract imaginative involvement with the demands of reality" (Gardner, 1974).

The basic determining factors of a child's hypnotic susceptibility have to do with the nature of their "child–adult experiences"; love and trust between parent and child; discipline techniques emphasizing firmness, consistency, and love orientation; and the presence of sibling relationships (an only child is less susceptible).

## Hypnotic Techniques

The following paragraphs describe the fundamental requirements of working hypnotically with children.

- Secure the child's attention. Entry into the child's world must be at his or her level, including use of fantasy and imagination, and the allowance for a shorter attention span.

- Formal induction (20 minutes). Somnambulistic suggestion – IV, story.

- Waking suggestion and semantics (30 seconds). Constant monologue with proper word choice and voice control (softer, quieter). Body language – smooth, gentle, slow movements, metronomic cadence to carotid pulse – tympanic membrane artery, NLP (Neurolinguistic Programming) – breathing and set-up of trigger point for relaxation. Distraction and sensory confusion – taste of anesthetic versus ice cream, rewards (toys), glove balloons. Needleless syringes should be used. The concurrent use of nitrous oxide etc. produces an altered state of consciousness similar to hypnosis, and facilitates and deepens normal and resistant subject induction.

*In Closing*
Again, no recipe was given for hypnotic induction because the technique must vary according to the professional, subject, situation, and objective.

Subliminal behavior modification for patient management and stress reduction is an important adjunct to practice.

# Dental Gagging

An overt or excessive gag reflex is usually a learned or conditional response – and thus, it can be unlearned (Zach, 1990).

Clarke and Pirsichetti (1988) report a case of a 51-year-old woman with a hypersensitive gag reflex. They developed the process of trance production while cooperating with the patient to develop her trances using her suggested images. An audiotape was made using those images with trays, mouthwash, and sponge to desensitize mouth and throat tissues, then using a denture base at home.

The salient elements of their approach with concurrent denture construction and desensitizing of a gag reflex were: (1) permissive hypnosis where the patient helps select hypnotic suggestions, (2) regular home practice of hypnorelaxation by the patient using tailor-made audiotapes, and (3) repeated rehearsal of planned procedures, for example, impressions. This attention to detail of dental treatment and desensitization of the gag reflex progressed concurrently, thus reducing the total time of treatment.

Wright (1979) investigated systemic causes of retching and found that, in general, evidence of greater incidence of gastrointestinal disorders or other systemic or social factors in retchers is lacking. In her study the only general health findings found to be significant were smoking and catarrh. Hypnopuncture – a combination treatment of hypnosis and acupuncture – provides a therapeutic treatment plan for long-term therapy for patients with a distinctive gag reflex. The treatment is applied independently of the cause. In cases of emergency treatment in dentistry, the immediate compliance of a patient is of utmost importance. The long-term goal of any therapeutic measure is control of the gag reflex. This new treatment protocol is illustrated in the case of a 50-year-old patient with a severe gag reflex presented by Eitner, Wichmann, and Holst (2005). After only five visits, dental treatment could be conducted without any auxiliary means. Hypnosis is applied in the form of hypnosedation (not as psychotherapy), while stereogenosis occupies a central position for desensitization.

Their case report as presented demonstrates the successful therapy of a severe gag reflex. The introduced concept of hypnopuncture combines the positive elements of hypnosis and acupuncture. Dental treatment can be carried out after two or three appointments. The long-term goal of hypnopuncture is the patient's (and dentist's) control of the gag reflex, not suppression. Patients experience their first "gag-free" dental appointment by the fourth or fifth visit. The basic principle is the application of hypnosedation in dentistry.

Barsby (1994) suggests that all of these techniques can be incorporated into the audiotape, which is then given to the patient on the second visit. The patient is instructed to use the tape at home, listening to it every day when the time and place are appropriate. Hypnosis is a useful aide in facilitating the management of patients with a "gagging" problem who have not previously been able to tolerate dentures. An eclectic approach is frequently successful. The reprogramming of patient attitudes and behavior may occasionally occur quite rapidly, but it can also be a slow process whereby patients are expected to learn self-hypnosis and to make use of audiotapes at home between visits. Essentially, the use of hypnosis allows patients a high level of autonomy and control over their treatment.

Sector, way back in 1952, demonstrates in a case report of severe gagging the advantages of continuity of care in general dentistry. He had seen a 44-year-old man many times from June 1947 to April 1952. Only one tooth was removed at each visit. Hypnosis was suggested to solve his dental problems, and he agreed to it. He entered into a fairly deep trance whereupon all remaining posterior teeth were removed. In October 1951, this man experienced a second hypnosis trance and two satisfactory impressions were made. In two subsequent visits, bite registration was taken and a try-in of wax dentures was made with the patient in induced deep trance. At the end of the same month, the rest of his teeth were removed without anesthesia. The dentures were inserted, adjusted, and seemed to be comfortable. Two days later the patient reported to the office. Remarkably rapid healing of the sites of the extractions was observed. The patient had worn the dentures constantly and was experiencing an abnormal increase in the salivary flow and occasional gagging. There were two sore areas due to peripheral overextension. The dentures were adjusted to relieve the areas of soreness. In trance it was suggested that this excess flow of saliva was useful only for digestion of abnormally large amounts of food that were not present. The suggestion was made to send to his brain the proper message and reduce the flow of saliva to normal. The excessive flow stopped. Then it was suggested that his occasional gagging was caused by the excess salivary flow and that since the flow was now normal the gagging would disappear entirely. He was seen on March 28, 1952 and he stated he was wearing his dentures at all times and was free of gagging. On his April 14, 1952, office visit, his teeth were loose and were causing gagging but he was able to wear the dentures. The dentures were rebased. In a phone call two weeks later, he reported neither discomfort nor gagging. The time required for the first induction was about 15 minutes. At this visit the posthypnotic suggestion was given that in the future he would enter the hypnotic state immediately on receiving a given signal. This suggestion was repeated at each visit. After the first induction the subsequent inductions required only a few seconds.

Morse, Hancock, and Cohen (1984) present a case report on *in vivo* desensitization using meditation-hypnosis in the treatment of tactile-induced gagging in a dental patient. This case is of interest for the following reasons: (1) It is the third reported case of the use of meditation-hypnosis technique for dentally related phobias, (2) meditation-hypnosis is an effective anti-anxiety agent for use in systematic desensitization, and it can be rapidly learned, (3) a long-standing gagging problem can be rapidly and effectively treated with mediation-hypnosis and systematic desensitization, and (4) the meditation-hypnosis technique is useful when generalized to other anxiety-inducing situations.

Weyandt (1972) presented three detailed cases in dental hypnotherapy. Hypnosis was the treatment of choice in the following three patients, two of whom were gaggers. The success of these three cases appears to be due to hypnotherapy plus strong individual motivation.

## Summary

The following outlines the salient features of gagging response – reasons, symptoms, patients, treatments, and hypnosis.

### Gagging
- Gut wrenching, wretched, retching.

- Purpose: To prevent foreign bodies from being inhaled into the lower airway. Gagging is a normal defense mechanism that protects the alimentary and respiratory tracts. The normal peristalsis of swallowing reverses in a spasmodic and uncoordinated fashion but ineffectual attempt to vomit.

- Symptoms: Extreme lacrimation; rhinorrhea; convulsive throat and abdomen; upper body and leg abduction; facial flushing; apnea; tachycardia; escape behavior, and exhaustion.

- Main trigger points in mouth for gag reflex are the fauces, uvula, and posterior pharyngeal wall.

- Causes: Neurogenic, physiologic, anatomic, iatrogenic, and metabolic.

- Iatrogenic: Impression of material dripping down throat, hard to remove dental appliance (traumatic removal). Near drowning, near suffocation, rape with orogenital penetration. Poor denture retention (especially maxillary), tissue coverage, occlusal errors of vertical and/or horizontal relationships, lack of space for tongue.

- Implant supported prostheses can eliminate postinsertion gagging problems.

## Patients

Most individuals who present for routine dental treatment with disruptive gagging are "mild retchers." Severe gaggers rarely present for routine dental treatment. Gagging is more prevalent in men than women. Fear is almost always the underlying factor influencing the psychological gagger.

Phobia is a severe psychological condition that dominates the patient's rationality. There is a behavioral tendency by the patient for protection from the perceived threat. An avoidance or escape from the threat and an emotional reaction of intense anxiety are prevalent – a set of conditions, obsessions, and relationships resulting in constant vigilance. The role of complex psychogenic or cognitive dental phobias is significant. Studies indicate approximately a 50% chance that a phobic will be highly responsive to hypnotic (suggestive) intervention.

Gaggers may not be effective at oral hygiene and could be at a greater risk of dental problems. One of the most serious problems affecting the patient with an overactive gag reflex is a strong potential for compromised treatment. In the dental environment, the patient may allow some procedures and be phobic of others but either way still perceives the overall dental experience as a threat.

## Treatment

It's essential to obtain a good history, especially concerning events that may have precipitated gagging episodes. If the short procedure is short, and a gag reflex mild, modifications to the procedure may suffice. Gaggers characteristically swallow with their teeth clenched and can be taught to modify this behavior to swallow with the teeth apart, tongue placed on hard palate, and orbicularis oris muscle relaxed. Simple relaxation approaches may be used, including progressive relaxation, basic stress reduction techniques, etc. Distraction, temporal tap, taping cheeks, and breathing similar to La Maze style may be helpful. Muscle stimulating activity, i.e., lifting leg, bending tongue blades, can be employed. Biofeedback pharmacological sedation, nitrous oxide, topical and local anesthetics, and table salt, are all options. Of course, pharmacological agents don't address the underlying psychological problem. Topical and local anesthetics are beneficial to the mild gagger.

## *Hypnosis*

All of the following are potentially helpful:

• Waking suggestion. Impression: Suggesting that something tasty is being placed in the mouth. Giving authoritarian commands and directions (eye contact, role playing). Imagery, i.e., breathing through imaginary hole in neck or numbed throat. Posthypnotic suggestions for increased comfort while wearing dentures. Hypnosis treatment should be followed by ego-strengthening and self-image improvement (magic mind mirror). Progressive desensitization is used for behavior modification to develop a coping response. Hypnosis and systematic desensitization are the treatment of choice for phobic gaggers.

## *References*

Abrahamsson, K. H. Berggren, U., Hallberg, L., & Carlsson, S. G. (2002). Dental phobic patients' view of dental anxiety and experiences in dental care: A qualitative study. *Scand J Caring Sci*, 16: 188–196.

Alladin, A. (2007). Evidence-based practice in clinical hypnosis. *Int J Clin Exp Hypn* Part I 55(2): 115–250, Part 11(3): 251–379.

Alladin, A., Sabatini, L., & Amundson, J. K. (2007). What should we mean by empirical validation in hypnotherapy: Evidence-based practice in clinical hypnosis. *Intl J Clin Exper Hypn* 55(2): 115–130.

Alman, B. M. & Lambrou, P. (1992). *Self-Hypnosis – The Complete Manual for Health and Self-Change* (2nd Edn). New York: Brunner/Mazel.

Barber, J. (1996). *Hypnosis and Suggestion in the Treatment of Pain – A Clinical Guide*. New York: W.W. Norton.

Barsby, M. J. (1994). The use of hypnosis in the management of "gagging" and intolerance of dentures. *Br Dent J*, 176: 97–102.

Bobart, V. & Brown, D. C. (2002). Medical obstetrical hypnosis and Apgar scores and the use of anaesthesia and analgesic during labor and delivery. *Hypnos* 29(3): 132–139.

Brown, D. C. & Hammond, D. C. (2007). Evidence-based clinical hypnosis in obstetrics, labor and delivery, and preterm labor. *Int J Clin Exper Hypn*, 55(3): 355–371.

Butler L. D., Symons, B. K., Henderson, S. L, Shortliffe, L. D., & Spiegel, D. (2005). Hypnosis reduces distress and duration of an invasive medical procedure for children. *Ped*, 115: e77–e85.

Canadian Medical Association Journal (1958). Miscellany: Hypnotism and medicine. *Can Med Ass J*, 78: 367–368.

Clarke, J. H. & Persichetti, S. J. (1988). Hypnosis and concurrent denture construction for a patient with a hypersensitive gag reflex. *Am J Clin Hypno*, 30: 285–288.

Crasilneck, H. B. & Hall, J. A. (1985). *Clinical Hypnosis – Principles and Applications* (2nd Edn). Boston: Allyn and Bacon.

Eitner, S., Schultze-Mosgau, S., Heckmann, J., Wichmann, M., & Holst, S. (2006). Changes in neurophysiologic parameters in a patient with dental anxiety by hypnosis during surgical treatment. *J Oral Rehab*, 33: 496–500.

Eitner, S., Wichmann, M. & Holst, S. (2005). A long term therapeutic treatment for patients with a severe gag reflex. *J of Clin and Exp Hyp*, 53(1): 74–86.

Elkins, G., Jensen, M. P. & Patterson, D. R. (2007). Hypnotherapy for the management of chronic pain. *Int J Clin Exp Hypn*, 55(3): 275–287.

Elliotson, J. (1843). Numerous cases of surgical operations without pain in the Mesmeric state. In D. N. Robinson (Ed.), *Significant Contributions to the History of Psychology 1750–1920*. Washington, DC: University Publications of America.

Erickson, M. H. & Rossi, E. L. (1979). *Hypnotherapy – An Exploratory Casebook*. New York: Irvington.

Ewin, D. M. & Eimer, B. (2006). Hypnotic preparation and core of the surgical patient. In *Idomotor Signs for Rapid Hypnoanaalysis: A How To Manual*. Springfield, IL: CC Thomas.

Fromm, E. & Nash, M. R. (1992). *Contemporary Hypnosis Research*. New York: Guildford.

Fromm, E. & Shor, R. E. (1979). *Hypnosis: Developments in Research and New Perspectives*. New York: Aldine.

Gardner, G. G. (1974). Hypnosis with children. *International Journal of Clinical and Experimental Hypnosis*, 22 (1): 20–28.

Gerschman, J. A. (1989). Hypnotizability and dental phobic disorders. *Anesthe Prog*, 36: 131–136.

Gerschman, J. A., Reade, P. C., & Burrows, G. D. (1980). Hypnosis in dentistry. In G. D. Burrows, & L. Dennerstein (Eds.), *Handbook of Hypnosis and Psychosomatic Medicine* (pp. 443–479). New York: Elsevier North Holland Press.

Gokli, M. A., Wood, A. J., Mourino, A. P., Farrington, F. H., & Best, A. M. (1994). Hypnosis as an adjunct to the administration of local anesthetic in pediatric patients. *J Dent Child*, July/Aug: 272–275.

Haley, J (1986). *Uncommon Therapy: The Psychiatric Techniques of Milton H. Erickson, MD*. New York: WW Norton.

Hammond D. C. (1990a). Suggestions in dental hypnosis. In D. C. Hammond (Ed.), *Handbook of Hypnotic Suggestions and Metaphors* (pp. 193–196). New York: W.W. Norton.

Hammond, D. C. (1990b). Review of the efficacy of clinical hypnosis with headaches and migraines. In D. C. Hammond (Ed.), *Handbook of Hypnotic Suggestions and Metaphors* (pp. 185–190). New York: W.W. Norton.

Havens, R. A. & Walters, C. (1989). *Hypnotherapy Scripts – A Neo-Ericksonian Approach to Persuasive Healing*. New York: Brunner/Mazel.

Hermes, D., Truebger, D., Hakim, S. G., & Sieg, P. (2004). Tape recorded hypnosis in oral and maxillofacial surgery – basic and first clinical experience. *J Cranio-Max Surg*, 33: 123–129.

Hilgard, E. R. (1965). *Hypnotic Susceptibility*. New York: Harcourt, Brace and World.

Hilgard, E. R., & Hilgard, J. R. (1975). *Hypnosis in the Relief of Pain*. Los Altos, CA: William Kauffman.

Hilgard, E. R. & Hilgard, J. R. (1994). Dentistry. In E. R. & J. R. Hilgard, *Hypnosis in the Relief of Pain* (Rev. Edn) (pp. 144–163). New York: Brunner/Mazel.

Hunter, M. (2004). *Understanding Dissociative Disorders. A Guide for Family Physicians and Health Care Professionals*. Carmarthen, Wales: Crown House Publishing Ltd.

Kuttner, L. (1991). Helpful strategies in working with preschool children in pediatric practice. *Pediatr Annals*, 20(3)/March: 120–127.

Kuttner, L. (2004). *A Child in Pain: How to Help, What to Do*. Leora Kuttner (distributed by Crown House Publishing, Bethel: Conn.)

Kvale, G., Berggren, U., & Milgrom, P. (2004). Dental fear in adults: A meta-analysis of behavioral interventions. *Com Dent Oral Epi*, 32: 250–264.

Lambert, S. A. (1996). The effects of hypnosis guided imagery on the postoperative course in children. *J Dev Behav Pediatr*, 17(2): 307–310.

Manusov, E. G. (1990). Clinical applications of hypnotherapy. *J. Fam Pract*, 31: 180–184.

Milling, L. S. & Constantino, C. A. (2000). Clinical hypnosis with children: First steps toward empirical support. *Int J Clin Exp Hypn*, 48(2): 113–137.

Montgomery, G. H., David, D., Winkel, G., Silverstein, J. H., & Bovbjerg, D. H. (2002). The effectiveness of adjunctive hypnosis with surgical patients: A meta-analysis. *Anesth Analg*, 94: 1639–1645.

Montgomery, G. H., DuHamel, K. N., & Redd, W. H. (2000). A meta-analysis of hypnotically induced analgesia: How effective is hypnosis? *Int J Clin Exp Hypn*, 48(2): 138–153.

Moore, R., Brodsgaard, I., & Abrahamsen, R. (2002). A three-year comparison of dental anxiety treatment outcomes: Hypnosis, group therapy and individual desensitization vs. no specialist treatment. *Eur J Oral Sci*, 110: 287–295.

Morse, D. R., Hancock, R. R., & Cohen, B. B. (1984). Case Report. In-vivo desensitization using meditation-hypnosis in the treatment of tactile-induced gagging in a dental patient. *Int J Psychosomatics*, 31: 20–23.

Nash, M. R. (2000). The status of hypnosis as an empirically validated clinical intervention. *Int J Clin Exp Hypn*, 48(2): 107–239.

Néron, S. & Stephenson, R. (2007). Effectiveness of hypnotherapy with cancer patients. *Int J Clin and Exp Hypn*, 55(3): 336–354.

O'Hanlon, W. H., & Martin, M. (1992). *Solution-Oriented Hypnosis – An Ericksonian Approach*. New York: W.W. Norton.

Olness, K. & Kohen, D. P. (1996). *Hypnosis and Hypnotherapy with Children* (3rd Edn). New York: Guilford.

Peretz, B. & Bimstein, E. (2000). The use of imagery suggestions during administration of local anesthetic in paediatric dental patients. *J Dent Chil*, 67(4): 263–267.

Rossi, E. L. (1993). *The Psychobiology of Mind–Body Healing – New Concepts of Therapeutic Hypnosis* (Rev Edn). New York: W.W. Norton.

Rustvold, S. R. (1994). Hypnotherapy for treatment of dental phobia in children. *Gen Dent* (July–Aug): 346–348.

Sector, I. I. (1952). Gagging controlled through hypnosis. *Dental Survey*, 28: 1366.

Scheflin, A. W. & Shapiro, J. L. (1989). *Trance on Trial*. New York: Guilford.

Shaw, A. J. & Welbury, R. R. (1996). The use of hypnosis in a sedation clinic for dental extractions in children: Report of 20 cases. *J Dent Chil*, 63: 418–420.

Spiegel, D. & Bloom J. R. (1983). Group therapy and hypnosis reduce metastatic breast carcinoma pain. *Psychosomatic Med*, 45(4): 333–339.

Spiegel, H. & Spiegel, D. (2004). *Trance and Treatment: Clinical Uses of Hypnosis.* Washington, DC: American Psychiatric Press.

Spiegel, L. J., & Peterson, L. (1980). Stress reduction in young dental patients through coping skills and sensory information. *J Consult Clin Psychol*, 48(6): 785–787.

Thompson, S. (1994). The use of hypnosis as an adjunct to nitrous oxide sedation in the treatment of dental anxiety. *Contemp Hypn*, 11(2): 77–83.

Weyandt, J. A. (1972). Three case reports in dental hypnotherapy. *Am J Clin Hypn*, 15(1): 49–55.

Wright, G. Z. (1975). *Behaviour Management in Dentistry for Children.* Philadelphia: Saunders.

Wright, S. M. (1979). An examination of factors associated with retching in dental patients. *J Dent*, 7: 194–207.

Yapko, M. D. (2003) *Trancework: An Introduction to the Practice of Clinical Hypnosis.* New York: Brunner-Routledge.

Zach, G. A. (1990). Hypnosis, Part III: Uses in dentistry. *Compend Contin Educ Dent*, XI(7): 420–425.

Zarren, J. I., & Eimer, B. N. (2002). *Brief Cognitive Hypnosis Facilitating the Change of Dysfunctional Behavior.* New York: Springer.

# Part III

# *Pain Management*

# Chapter 9

# Hypnosis, Anesthesiology, and Pain

*A. Max Chaumette*

## Introduction

This chapter covers hypnosis and anesthesiology in the perioperative period and in the management of chronic pain.

My interest in hypnosis began in earnest with my involvement in the treatment of chronic pain. A young woman came to our clinic after failure of the classical treatment for migraines on her left side. I felt powerless because all the medical options that I knew of at the time had been exhausted. I consulted with one of my colleagues. Upon hearing of my predicament, she took a cassette tape from the library and placed a temperature probe on the patient's left finger and played the cassette tape. While seated, the patient listened to the words from the cassette player. In awe, I witnessed the changes in the facial expressions of the patient and was astonished to notice a steady rise in the temperature of her monitored finger. The temperature of her finger returned to normal when the tape was finished and her symptoms disappeared. The ability to use carefully chosen words to elicit physiological changes intrigued me and I decided to learn hypnosis.

## Historical Overview of Hypnosis

The phenomenon of hypnosis has been known for ages in all cultures. The beginning of modern hypnosis is generally attributed to the work of Dr. Franz Anton Mesmer (1734–1815). Living in France in 1784, Mesmer had multiple encounters with a street hypnotist who used magnets. Mesmer came to believe that the magnets had a power of their own to correct medical problems and bring back good health. He eventually coined the term of *animal magnetism*. It seemed that certain patients entered a state of stupor and apparently all signs of illness disappeared.

Mesmer also recognized the importance of rapport and was probably the first Western physician to use psychotherapy as a concept. Benjamin Franklin (1706–1790), then ambassador to France, watched the work of Mesmer and with Joseph Guillotin (1738–1814) and Antoine Lavoisier (1743–1794) concluded that imagination played a significant role in the results. As a result, Mesmer became discredited and the study of mesmerism went underground.

In 1824, Professor John Elliotson (1792–1888) of the University of London reported on numerous cases of surgical operations without pain during the mesmeric state. One of his disciples, the Scottish physician, James Esdaille (1808–1859) went to India where he enjoyed more freedom to operate on Indians. Between 1840 and 1850, Esdaille preformed more than 1,000 minor and 345 major operations using "mesmerism" as the sole anesthetic agent. His morbidity and mortality rate was 5%, while for all other surgeons of that era it was hovering around 50%. It was a remarkable feat because antibiotics and modern anesthesia were unknown at the time. These surgeries included excision of 14 scrotal tumors weighing from 8 to 80 pounds, amputations, and mastectomies for cancer. Esdaille hoped the new technique would become widely available and accepted.

On Thursday, October 16, 1846, before Esdaille's book could be published, William Morton, a Boston dentist administered diethyl ether to Gilbert Abbot. Harvard surgeon John Collins Warren, who had prior experience with hypnotic anesthesia, removed a tumor from Abbot's neck without the patient showing any sign of pain or awareness of the procedure. The news spread fast. This experiment with ether was repeated in Paris and in London. In December 1846, as reported by Hilgard and Hilgard (1975), Robert Liston proclaimed: "Gentlemen, this is no humbug; the Yankee dodge beat the mesmerism hollow."

By 1848, ether, nitrous oxide, chloroform, and other chemical agents were widely used in dentistry, surgery, and obstetrics. This resulted in a decline in the use of hypnosis for surgical, dental, and obstetrical interventions especially once Queen Victoria received general anesthesia with chloroform while giving birth to her last child, Prince Leopold. According to Hilgard and Hilgard (1994), general anesthesia was then described by medical practitioners of the time as "inevitable, safe and complete." It became an accepted and approved medical modality. Hypnotism, as applied to surgical interventions, was relegated to a dustbin of history. Hypnosis moved primarily into the sphere of psychotherapy.

Fast forward to the beginning of the twentieth century. Dr. Henry Monro of Omaha, Nebraska, strongly believed in preparing patients for surgery to diminish the anxiety and apprehension associated with a surgical intervention. After putting his patients in a hypnotic state, he would discuss their misgivings, fears, and would conclude by telling them that they would recover promptly after the operation and that they would feel great. Dr. Monro discovered that following hypnosis sessions, only 25% of ether was needed to produce a satisfactory anesthesia and that recovery was fast and unremarkable. Following his intuition, he repeated the procedure with over 100 consecutive surgical patients and concluded that whenever he used hypnosis, only 10–25% of the expected amount of ether was necessary to achieve satisfactory results. He was ridiculed by other physicians until he talked to William and Charles Mayo.

In Rochester, Minnesota, the Mayo brothers also followed their curious instincts and experimented with this new technique for their surgical patients. They performed 17,000 abdominal cases without an anesthetic, death or injury. The whole world focused its attention on the Mayo clinic. Alice Magaw, the nurse anesthetist who administered many of these anesthetics, wrote in the *Journal of Surgery, Gynecology and Obstetrics* in December 1906: "By employment of suggestion scientifically and earnestly, very little ether is required to produce surgical anesthesia, even less chloroform to keep a patient surgically anesthetized."

Nonetheless, not enough weight was given to those words and for about 40 years, the use of hypnosis in anesthesiology went into decline. However, in the late 1950s, hypnosis experienced a revival and several physicians, including anesthesiologists, made some valuable contributions:

- R. V. August, M.D., described the preparation necessary for the use of hypnosis as the sole agent for anesthesia. He filmed a patient undergoing a caesarian using hypnosis as the sole agent of anesthesia.

- Andrew Saint Amand, M.D., described the phenomenon of "voodoo death" after investigating the death of several individuals who predicted their deaths at a specific time and whose autopsies failed to reveal any organic disorder. Because of his work, we take seriously any patient who mentions during the perioperative period the possibility of dying. In fact, when a patient thinks that he or she may die, and there is no effective way to convince the person otherwise, the surgery should be cancelled and psychological or psychiatric help should be provided before returning the patient to the surgical area.

- Bertha Rodger, M.D., stressed the importance of suggestions in the immediate preoperative period and the need to speak to patients during the administration of general anesthesia and upon reaching the postoperative area.

- David Cheek, M.D., used ideomotor signals to prove conclusively that patients can and do hear under general anesthesia. He also used hypnosis as a sole anesthetic agent.

- Dabney Ewin, M.D., discovered the conditions that enable hearing under anesthesia. He also described the characteristics of the patient that can tolerate hypnosis as the sole anesthetic agent.

- Robert Pearson, M.D., proved that the hospital stay of patients who listened to a recorded message suggesting a shorter postoperative stay were discharged by an average of 2.42 days earlier than patients who did not listen to that message.

- Christel Bejenke, M.D., presented several lectures on hypnosis and anesthesiology introducing many to this discipline.

- Lillian Fredericks, M.D., wrote in 2000 a much-needed and well-received text, *The Use of Hypnosis in Surgery and Anesthesiology*. This comprehensive text outlines in detail the role that hypnosis must play in the practice of anesthesiology.

## *Practical Considerations*

I am no longer familiar with the surgical practices in Canada. When I think of the practice of anesthesiology today in the United States, I cannot help but express some feelings of longing for the *good old days* prior to managed care.

Prior to managed care, when a patient was scheduled for a surgical intervention, he or she was admitted to the hospital on the eve of the surgical date. It was pleasant to review leisurely the patient's chart to note salient data of history, physical findings, and laboratory studies. Following this, I would go to the patient's room for the pre-op visit and assess the patient's attitude toward the surgery scheduled for the following day. This pre-op visit gave the patient an opportunity to freely express fears, worries, and hopes. During this visit, I would also fully explain to the patient what he or she could expect once wheeled into the operating room theater.

Nowadays, for an elective surgery, the patient is seen by somebody who may or may not be the individual who will administer the anesthetic. This rapport cannot be transmitted to the physician who will finally administer the anesthetic. Because of time constraints, the anesthesiologist quickly reviews the chart and talks to the patient to become familiar with the personality and wishes of the patient. This conversation with the patient is critical for patient and anesthesiologist to establish a meaningful rapport.

This is how I usually approach a patient:

After checking for a signed informed consent, I tell the patient: "Good morning! I am Dr. Chaumette. I am going to be in charge of your anesthesia. I have reviewed your chart and everything seems to be in order. Do you have any question that I should address? Here is the procedure that I will follow..." And then describe in detail the induction, maintenance, and emergence of the anesthesia without omitting any detail regarding the possibility of blood loss, nausea, vomiting, pain, and the need to breathe deeply and ambulate when asked to by the nursing personnel.

All of these details are necessary because anesthesiology is an entirely referred practice. Here is what usually happens prior to an operation. The patient first sees a family practitioner followed perhaps by an internist prior to being referred to a surgeon. While visiting all those physicians, the patient has a chance to develop a rapport with them. When the day of surgery arrives, the patient meets a new face: the anesthesiologist, assigned just by luck to the case. The anesthesiologist is responsible for taking away the patient's elementary faculties and ability to remain conscious. The time to develop a rapport with the patient is too limited. The patient has no time to check the credentials of the anesthesiologist. This atmosphere contributes to the patient's anxiety.

Therefore, it is very important to be attentive to the state of mind of the patient prior to surgery. In order to reduce the likelihood of related complications, here is a list of some things to avoid:

1. *I am going to put you to sleep.* In North America, pets at the end of their lives are put to sleep and never recover. The patient may have gone through such an experience and the subconscious may misunderstand and misinterpret the words so spoken.

2. *Try.* The word *try* implies the possibility of failure. One should have an upbeat attitude when talking to a patient.

3. *Lie.* We should always be factual. There is a way to inform a patient of bad news while being upbeat and factual. For example, one should tell a patient that the success rate is about 20% and that one feels that the patient will be one of the 20%.

4. *Pain.* It is wise to talk only of comfort or discomfort when starting an intravenous perfusion. It is better to tell the patient: "I am not sure how much this may bother you; since you are able to control any discomfort, you will probably be happily surprised when you discover that it does not bother you as much as you first thought."

5.  *It is all over* or *You are finished* or *Let's get out of here*. When a person of authority (anesthesiologist, surgeon, and nurse in charge) uses those words, the subconscious takes things literally and the patient may have some adverse inexplicable and unexpected physiological changes, i.e., sudden rise in heart rate and blood pressure.

# Hypnosis Management during Anesthesia Administration

## Preinduction

A formal hypnosis session prior to induction of anesthesia is not always necessary. An appropriate message to the patient contributes to good results: decreased blood loss, post-op analgesia, absence of nausea and vomiting. My personal preference is to have a formal session of hypnosis. In such cases, I always request the presence of a witness such as a nurse or family member. Because of time constraints, I have developed a brief session, the text of which is presented later in this chapter.

## Induction

Upon starting an intravenous perfusion, the word "pain" should never be used when talking to the patient. Let's assume that the current patient is female. Generally, I ask the patient to breathe slowly and that my touching will not bother her at all. I inform the patient of what to expect from the anesthesiology. I cover all the stages from induction to recovery. I encourage the patient to express any feeling that she may experience as we speak. I create an environment that allows the patient to understand our partnership during the perioperative period. When the patient is wheeled into the surgical suite, I continue to give some encouraging words.

When the induction begins, I ask the patient to go into her mind in the most pleasant place of her choice. I then tell her that soon she will enjoy a pleasant snooze. I continue to communicate with the patient during the whole induction process. Even when the patient is asleep, I continue to inform her of all my actions step by step. I make a point of telling the patient when I insert an endotracheal tube to facilitate ventilation during the surgical procedure.

## Maintenance

During the operation, I either put earphones on the patient playing soothing music (the patient's taste and preference must always be considered) while the procedure is in progress or I continue to reassure the patient using a message similar to the preinduction session that is described later.

I tell the patient to remain in good spirits, that blood loss should be minimal and that discomfort, if any, should be minimal. Talking to the patient during the procedure is critical since I share the opinion that patients can hear while under general anesthesia. And because I have no control over the conversation between the other members of the surgical team, I maintain verbal contact with the patient throughout the surgery. This is one of the best ways to protect a patient from hearing words that may be poorly understood while the procedure is in progress. This process enables me to preserve the healing environment carefully created during the pre-op visit.

## Emergence and Recovery

When the patient wakes up from the anesthesia, I inform her that all went well and that recovery will happen faster than expected. It is important to maintain an encouraging atmosphere. I strongly discourage the use of negative ideas. In the recovery room, the patient receives a detailed description of her condition. This enables the recovery to be smooth and rapid.

To avoid any suggestion of emesis, all emesis basins are kept as far away as possible. I encourage the patient to return to the pleasant place where she went during the induction and enjoy it. Such an approach reduces the need for pain medication.

In my experience, patients who are prepared hypnotically recover much faster and need less pain medication. The incidence of nausea and vomiting is nil. The recovery of all body functions is rapid and emergence delirium is very rare.

## Summary

In summary, hypnosis in the perioperative period helps decrease anxiety and apprehension associated with the anticipated anesthesia and surgery. It enables the patient to cooperate better with the surgical team. It also potentiates the effect of all chemical agents used during the administration of anesthesia, thus reducing the dosage necessary to obtain therapeutic effects. Blood loss is reduced to a minimum.

In the postoperative period, emergence delirium is very rare; if a little discomfort exists, it is easily tolerated. This results in a decreased need for any medication. An early return to normal bladder and bowel functions is observed. When no contraindication exists, appetite also returns early; the immune system is stimulated, healing begins immediately, and recovery time is shortened. The postoperative course is smoother than expected.

## *Hypnosis Script Prior to Anesthesia Induction: Sample Text*

Are you as comfortable as you can be? If not, make yourself as comfortable as possible. As you do so, please take a few long, slow deep breaths and exhale slowly and enjoy the relaxation that this activity triggers. See how good you feel? Allow your eyes to close as you relax your eye muscles to the point that they will not work. That's right! When that happens, test them and make sure that they do not work and enjoy the relaxation that spreads from your head to your toes without missing a square inch. That's right! Your head, neck, arms, chest are relaxing more and more, so are your abdomen, pelvis, legs and feet. That's right! In fact you are so relaxed that you may right now see yourself on the fifth floor of a building where you are soon going to walk down to the first floor. That's right! As you descend, you happily discover that as you change floors, your level of relaxation increases by leaps and bounds. That's right! Going down and down reaching the fourth floor where you enjoy ten times more relaxation. That's right! Going down and down again and as you reach the third floor, you find yourself twenty times more relaxed. That's right! Going down and down reaching the second floor relaxing more and reaching the first floor where you enjoy a state of absolute relaxation. That's right! This state of relaxation enables you to see yourself in a wonderful place of special beauty where you enjoy sounds, lights, colors, tastes, feel and smell. Everything around you seems so perfect. That's right! You are basking in happiness and you feel that there is nothing to bother you as you enjoy complete comfort, peace and safety. That's right!

Your surgeon and you have agreed that you need this surgical intervention. I will administer the anesthesia that is necessary to enable the surgical team to perform the procedure to the best of its ability. I will remain with you as long as need be, watching you and making sure that you remain safe and comfortable. That's right! You may hear me talk to you and you will only pay attention to my voice. And, once the operation begins and until it is finished, you will keep all your blood. That's right! At the end of the procedure, you will awaken as if you just enjoyed a very restful, peaceful sleep, feeling great, refreshed and alert. The ease with which you follow the orders of the recovery room team will amaze all. You may be happily surprised when you discover how well everything goes during and after the operation and you experience much less need for medication of any kind during and after the procedure; furthermore, you will be up and about and will experience the return of all body functions to a normal condition (good appetite, breathing deeply, walking, moving bowels and urinating) and you will heal much earlier than all expect enabling you to have a very short hospital stay. That's right!

Now, I am soon going to leave you with these beautiful thoughts. I will shortly facilitate your orientation to here and now. I will count from one to five to allow you to re-alert yourself at your own pace to enable you to obtain a great feeling of ease and comfort. One, feeling good and great. Two, enjoying your newfound sensation of well-being. Three, knowing that you will be just fine. Four, enjoying your relaxation more and becoming more and more alert, being able to go back to this beautiful place at will. Five, reoriented to here and now and being able to enjoy so much safety, comfort and peace. That's good! That's excellent!

## Hypnosis and Pain Management

In 1979, the International Association for the Study of Pain stated that:

> Pain is an unpleasant sensory and emotional experience associated with actual or potential tissue damage.

Pain is either *acute* or *chronic*.

Acute pain is a symptom that indicates an injury and the reaction to that injury. Anxiety and signs of sympathetic discharge are noticed: tachycardia, hypertension, and increased perspiration. The treatment modality should include treatment of anxiety. One such method is to invite patients to go to their "laughing place" as described by Dabney Ewin, M.D. in his seminars.

Chronic pain is a syndrome dominated by symptoms lasting longer than six months. Signs of depression occur including sleep and appetite disturbances, irritability, social withdrawal, decreased pain tolerance, and constipation.

The psychological factors dominate so much that S. Weir Mitchell stated in 1872: "Perhaps few persons who are not physicians can realize the influence which long, continued and unendurable pain may have upon both body and mood."

When a patient complains of chronic pain, the clinician should first investigate the cause. Sometimes a disease presents itself with pain as the first symptom. Often, there are no objective findings; the physical examination and lab work are within normal limits. Evaluation of the patient must include psychological and physical examination on equal footing.

Generally, a patient with chronic pain has been under the care of several clinicians or physicians for an extended period. Therefore, it is important not to be complacent. It is also critical to listen carefully to the patient so as not to mistakenly assume that it is just the same old symptoms that need no further evaluation and possibly err in the diagnosis and treatment.

During the first visit, the pain specialist must establish a good rapport with the patient. Gaining the confidence and full cooperation of the patient are critical to achieve the best possible results. For example, doctors universally wear white coats. Since doing pain work, I have made it a habit to wear only light blue lab coats. In so doing, I aim to communicate to patients that we are partners in their treatment.

The chronic pain patient has been around many practitioners and some have said that the problem is in his or her head, adding that nothing can be done with the pain and that the patient must learn to live with it. The challenge for the pain specialist is to convince the patient that everything possible will be undertaken to help and that he or she will be treated as an individual. Accordingly, a full understanding of the condition is useful to both patient and physician. A caring attitude, good manners, consideration, and respect help create an atmosphere where positive results are possible.

The physician must inform the patient of all steps in the evaluation and management of the patient's condition. This may be tedious, but the physician must reassure the patient at every step of that undertaking.

The physician must review all previous diagnoses and treatments. It may not be unusual to find that a previous diagnosis had no bearing on the condition or complaints. Whether or not a previous diagnosis is found to be correct, a full investigation must follow. Prior to deciding on a treatment modality, previous psychological evaluations, treatments, and consultations with all other specialists must also be taken into consideration.

The medical history of the patient must be complete and thorough. While taking the history, the physician must often express eagerness to help and visibly show deep interest in the patient's condition. The presence of a patient's spouse or significant other under some circumstances can help in the process of obtaining an accurate history.

The medical history must be recorded clearly and in a methodical manner. First, the patient describes the reason for the current visit. While taking the history, the physician must observe and note the patient's appearance (grooming), manners, gestures, behavior, and emotional reactions. Listening carefully and attentively to what the patient says and how it is said enables the physician to have a more complete picture as well as determine whether or not the patient has an ulterior motive (such as financial compensation) or is mentally imbalanced.

## Medical History

A detailed description of the general health of the patient prior to the onset of pain should be recorded. Prior accidents, periods of disabilities, diseases, and injuries should be part of the inquiry. This information will be used to determine what pain management is applicable. This enables the physician to avoid using a treatment modality that has provided no relief to the patient in the past.

## Family History

The physician must make a tactful inquiry about the health of parents and siblings. It is always useful to know if any other member of the family experienced frequent painful disorders and periods of disability. Furthermore, the physician should also determine whether the patient was abused as a child because chronic pain could be a distant result of that prior experience.

## Psychological History

A psychological evaluation may reveal signs of depression manifested by sleep and appetite disturbances, irritability, social withdrawal, and constipation.

## Location of Pain

Location of pain is important. It is best evaluated while the symptom is present because when it ceases, the accuracy of the site description may not be reliable.

- Localized pain exists whenever the symptom is confined to the site of origin without any radiation.

- Projected pain is felt as if transmitted along the course of a nerve.

- Referred pain is experienced far from the source of the current problem along same segment.

- Reflex sympathetic dystrophy does not follow any segmental or peripheral nerve distribution.

- Psychological pain does not fit any anatomical pattern and may involve the whole body or various pains scattered throughout the body.

## Quality of Pain

The physician should ask whether the pain is sharp, burning, dull, diffuse, localized.

## Severity of Pain

Pain is very subjective. The best way is to ask the patient to rate his or her pain level on a scale of 0–10; 0 meaning no pain and 10 meaning it is absolutely intolerable.

## Duration of Pain

The physician should ask whether the pain is intermittent, continuous, pulsing, or like a wave, increasing and decreasing in intensity.

## Physical Examination

A thorough review of all prior treatment received by the patient and a complete physical examination are of utmost importance. It is essential to remember that the complaint of pain might mask serious problems. For example, "headaches" could indicate the presence of a brain tumor or an aneurysm or an AV malformation. All of this information is contained in the Chronic Pain Assessment form (at the end of this chapter) that the patient is asked to complete. Finally, the physician explains to the patient the hypnosis treatment modality.

## Treatment

The treatment of chronic pain is very complex. It involves the cooperation of practitioners of several disciplines such as: internal medicine, psychiatry, psychology, social work, anesthesiology, neurology, and neurosurgery. The role of the psychologist and social worker is to create a climate where the patient can tolerate the pain. Support groups for pain patients are invaluable. The role of the other specialists is self-evident. From an anesthesiology point of view, whenever the pain is localized or follows the path of a nerve, or if RSD (reflex sympathetic dystrophy) is present, blocks may be offered to the patient. In my 25-year experience, the combination of a local anesthetic drug and a narcotic potentiated the analgesia provided by an epidural or subarachnoid block without worry of relative overdose of either agent. While inserting the blocks, the hypnotic message given to the patient often decreases the dosage needed to achieve analgesia.

Whenever the pain is generalized, it is not feasible to offer a block to the patient, because no nerve roots are identified. Hypnosis is therefore a desirable treatment modality in such a case.

## Hypnotic Techniques

After establishing a satisfactory rapport with the patient, the hypnosis session may begin. According to Harold Crasilneck, Ph.D. (1985) patients with chronic pain syndrome are usually great subjects. Several methods can be used to hypnotize them.

I usually like to dissociate patients by asking them after induction to go to a very special place of their choosing where all their senses are stimulated. While they enjoy the ambiance, I ask them to see a rheostat attached to the center of the brain responsible for the symptom(s) that the patient experiences. I never use the word pain, preferring to use the word *discomfort*. The dial of the rheostat shows the same number as the pain level indicated on the Chronic Pain Assessment form that the patient previously filled out. Ideomotor signaling is used to verify all perceptions of the patient; the patient is then asked to decrease slowly and progressively the number on the rheostat to a comfortable level. Ideomotor signaling must validate the realization of such goals.

Another approach is to suggest to the patient to see all shades of the pain color disappearing to yield in their place his or her favorite color. A variation of this technique is to suggest that the patient sees the shape of the pain (without ever using that word) and slowly have that shape transformed to the one that means absence of pain. All those results are validated with ideomotor signaling. Unless there is resistance, the ideomotor signaling enables the physician to gauge the progress of the session.

As described by Hilgard and Hilgard (1975), sometimes a "hidden observer" is added to enhance the ability of the patient to diminish the number on the screen or rheostat and also strengthen his or her ego. This method enables the patient to function without being psychologically attached to the care provider. A self given cue such as pressing two fingers together when the comfortable number is reached allows the patient to eliminate the unpleasant sensations at will.

When I first began to work in hypnosis with pain patients, I used to count backwards beginning with the number of the pain level to deepen the hypnotic state. At emergence, I would count forward to the same number. Working with a patient, I learned that counting forward to the same number can induce the return of unpleasant symptoms. I have since abandoned that method of emergence in pain patients. Instead, I congratulate them for a job well done and ask them to return to a state of alertness fully oriented to place and time.

As a rule, I record the hypnosis session on an audio or video cassette. Sometimes, I give a copy of the audio cassette to the patient advising him to listen to it whenever a refresher is needed. I also warn the patient not to drive nor operate any electrical or mechanical devices while listening to the tape. When I give the tape to the patient, I usually add that I do not expect that the patient will find it necessary to listen to the cassette because the patient was a great subject.

According to Harold Crasilneck (1985), hypnosis should be offered to chronic pain patients because so many of them are helped when the hypnosis session is done properly. I share this opinion.

## Hypnosis as the Sole Anesthetic Agent

As mentioned earlier, Dr. James Esdaille performed hundreds of surgeries minor and major using hypnosis as the sole anesthetic agent, in India in the early 1840s, and his morbidity and mortality were about 5% compared to the norm of 50%± of the time. In 1958, Dr. Marmer reported doing major thoracic surgeries on very sick patients using hypnosis as the sole anesthetic.

I saw a film in which Dr. R. V. August was involved in the caesarian section on a patient done with hypnosis as the sole agent. That was in 1960, the same year in which Dr. Maurice Tinterow described using hypnosis as the sole agent for the cholecystectomy of his secretary. In 1980, Dr. Victor Rausch of Toronto, Ontario, used self-hypnosis as the sole agent for his cholecystectomy. Dr. David Cheek used hypnosis twice as the sole agent. The medical literature contains several such examples.

While undergoing a surgical intervention under hypnosis as the sole agent, patients may deny any distress and discomfort while showing signs of sympathetic discharge (hypertension, tachycardia, heavy perspiration, frowning). Whenever those signs appear, chemical anesthesia may be administered. But often times, many patients show no sign of distress.

According to Dr. Dabney Ewin, those who tolerate hypnosis as the sole agent share the following characteristics:

1.  They are motivated;

2.  They believe that they can use hypnosis as sole agent and they experience a need sometimes because of their general health;

3.  They need the operation.

Hypnosis as the sole anesthetic agent should not be offered to most patients because it is not always successful. The patient's preparation consumes a lot of time and rehearsals are very tedious. In this era of managed care such preparation is not always economically feasible. Furthermore, in the opinion of Dr. William Kroger (1977), only 10% of the general population may be able to undergo hypno-anesthesia when chemical anesthesia is available. Despite these variables, the hypnotist must always exude confidence to the patient lest his or her doubts trigger some negative thoughts or some misgivings in the patient which could lead to complete failure of that undertaking.

## Conclusion

Recognized as a treatment modality by the American Medical Association since 1958, the medical profession has taken too long to integrate hypnosis into daily practice. I firmly believe that hypnosis should become an integral part of the anesthesiology practice. All anesthesiology residency programs should include the teaching of hypnosis in their curriculum.

# Chronic Pain Assessment

### A. Max Chaumette, Jr., M.D., ABMH
Mchaumette@aol.com

Date _____

Name _____Birth date_____ Age _____

Address _____

_____

City, State, Zip _____

Phone _____

Occupation _____

Name and address of Employer

_____

_____

Present work status _____Phone_____

Years of Schooling

_____

Marital Status *(Single, engaged, separated, married, divorced, living together, widowed, other)*

_____

Describe current relationship

_____

Previous diagnoses, consultations, treatments and outcomes

_____

_____

_____

History of current problem:

_____

_____

_____

Past and present medications include: *(list medication, dosage, frequency, effectiveness, and reason for discontinuing)*

_____

_____

_____

Smoking _____ Coffee _____ Tea _____ Alcohol _____ (Cocaine, marijuana, amphetamines, other)

_____

What triggers or improves your symptoms *(circle the words that best describe your answer)*?

Worry, tension, physical activity, menstrual cycle, relaxation, weekends, vacations, work, reading, concentration, studying, attending lectures, noises, excitement, spats, anger, emotional times, hot baths, sunshine, precision work, sexual activity, annoyances, certain foods, fatigue, alcohol, weather, sympathy, attention, or other?

_____

By what percentage have the following activities been adversely affected by your problems:

Leisure _____ Social activity _____ Sexual activity _____ Sleep _____

House chores _____ Appetite _____ Relationships _____ Daily routine _____

Weight gain (lbs _____ Weight loss (lbs) _____ Fatigue _____

Poor concentration _____ Guilt feelings _____ Loss of sexual interest _____

Irritability _____ Suicide thoughts _____

How do people who live with you know you are in pain?

_____

Reaction of family to your pain *(circle the words that best describe your answer)*:

Ignore, angry, detached, supportive, encouragement to be active, other

_____

_____

On a scale of one to ten, where one is no pain and ten is the worst pain you could ever imagine anyone ever having, how would you rate your pain?

_____

What is your favorite color? What is the color of your pain? What color is the absence of pain

_____

What is the shape of your pain? What shape is the absence of pain?

_____

Describe your pain *(circle the words that best describe your answer)*:

Splitting, dull, crushing, throbbing, cramping, stabbing, tingling, sore, burning, shouting, pins and needles or other

_____

Describe the intensity of your pain *(circle the words that best describe your answer)*:

ongoing/constant, variable/change over time, comes and goes or other

_____

_____

_____

If your pain comes and goes, does it begin and finish at the same time daily?

_____

Where do you experience the most pain?

_____

_____

_____

What difference would it make in your life if suddenly you had no pain?

_____

_____

Do you want to get better?

_____

What pain level reduction would satisfy you?

_____

Are you willing to work with me to improve your symptoms?

_____

What do you like the most about yourself?

_____

_____

What do you dislike about yourself?

_____

_____

What else do you feel I need to know about you and your condition?

_____

_____

_____

Signature of Patient _____

# *Bibliography*

August, R. V. (1960). Obstetric hypnoanesthesia. *American Journal of Obstetrics and Gynecology*, 79, 1131–1138.

Barber, J. (1996). *Hypnosis and Suggestion in the Treatment of Pain: A Clinical Guide*. New York: W.W. Norton.

Burrows, G. D., & Dennerstein, L. (Eds.) (1980). *Hypnosis and Psychosomatic Medicine*. New York: Elsevier/North Holland Biomedical Press.

Cheek, D. B. (1994). *Hypnosis: The Application of Ideomotor Techniques*. Boston: Allyn and Bacon.

Crasilneck, H. B. & Hall, J. (1985). *Clinical Hypnosis: Principles and Applications* (2nd edn). Boston: Allyn and Bacon.

Druckman, D., & Bjork, R. A. (Eds.) (1992). *In the Mind's Eye: Enhancing Human Performance*. Washington DC: National Academy Press. Additional Author: National Research Council (US) Committee on Techniques for the Enhancement of Human Performance.

Elliotson, J. (1843/1977). *Numerous Cases of Surgical Operations Without Pain in the Mesmeric State* (Vol. 10). Washington, DC: University Publications of America.

Esdaile, J. (1846/1977). *Mesmerism in India, and its Practical Application in Surgery and Medicine* (Vol. 10). Washington, DC: University Publications of America.

Ewin, D. M. (1998). Rapid eye roll induction. In: D. C. Hammond (Ed.), *Hypnotic Induction and Suggestion*. New York: W.W. Norton.

Fredericks, L. E. (2000). *The Use of Hypnosis in Surgery and Anesthesiology*. Springfield, IL: Charles C. Thomas.

Hammond, D. C. (Ed.) (1990). *Hypnotic Suggestions and Metaphors*. New York: W.W. Norton.

Hilgard, E. R. & Hilgard, J. (1975). *Hypnosis in the Relief of Pain*. Los Altos, CA: Kaufman

Kroger, W. (1977). Clinical and experimental hypnosis. *Medical and Dental and Psychology Series* (2nd edn). Philadelphia: Lippincott Co.

Magaw, A. (1906). A review of over fourteen thousand surgical anesthesias. *Journal of Surgery, Gynecology and Obstetrics*, 3(6), 795–799.

Marmer, M. J. (1958). The hypnotized heart. *Time Magazine*.

Meyer, R. G. (1992). Practical clinical hypnosis, techniques and applications. In *Scientific Foundations of Clinical Counseling Psychology*. New York: Lexington Books.

Mitchell, S. W. (1872). *Injuries of Nerves and their Consequences*. Self-published monograph.

Pearson, R. E. P. (1961). Response to suggestions given under general anesthesia. *American Journal of Clinical Hypnosis*, 4, 106–114.

Pearson, R. E. P. (1973). Why doesn't it work for me? The 16th Annual Meeting of the American Society of Clinical Hypnosis. Toronto, Canada.

Rodger, B. (1961). The art of preparing the patient for anesthesia. *Anesthesiology*, 22, 548.

Rodger, B. (1962). Hypnosis in anesthesia: Some psychological considerations. *American Journal of Clinical Hypnosis*, 4, 237.

Rodger, B. (1964). Recognition and use of hypnoidal behavior in the surgical patient. *American Journal of Clinical Hypnosis*, 6, 355.

Rossi, E., & Cheek, D. (1994). *Mind–body Therapy: Methods of Ideodynamic Healing in Hypnosis*. New York: W.W. Norton.

Tinterow, M. M. (1960). The use of hypnotic anesthesia for a major surgical procedure. *American Surgery*, 26, 732–737.

Wester, W. C. II (1987). *Clinical Hypnosis: A Case Management Approach*. Cincinnati, OH: Behavioral Sciences Center.

Wester, W. C. II, & Smith, A. H. (Eds.) (1984). *Clinical Hypnosis: A Multidisciplinary Approach*. Philadelphia: Lippincott.

White, J. C., & Sweet, W. H. (Eds.) (1955). *Pain: Its Mechanism and Neurosurgical Control*. Springfield, IL: Charles C. Thomas.

Zilbergeld, B., Edelstein, M. G., & Araoz, D. L. (Eds.) (1986). *Hypnosis, Questions and Answers*. New York: W.W. Norton.

## Chapter 10

# Resolving Traumatic Memories Related to Persistent and Recurring Pain

*James H. Straub and Vicki W. Straub*

Traumatic memories and post-traumatic stress disorder (PTSD) are often related to persistent pain, anxiety and other difficulties seen in medical, surgical and dental procedures and treatment. In addition to physical injuries resulting from trauma, a variety of pain-related syndromes are significantly correlated with a history of PTSD (Shipherd, Keyes, et al., 2007; Villano, Rosenblum, et al., 2007; Andreski, Chilcoat, & Breslau, 1998; Asmundson & Taylor, 2006; Geisser, Roth, et al., 1996; Otis, Pincus, et al., 2006; Santos, 1997). A significant number of women with chronic pelvic pain have experienced sexual or physical abuse (Heim, Ehlert, et al., 1998; Lampe, Solder, et al., 2000). Engel (2003) looked at the relationship between multiple idiopathic physical symptoms (MIPS) and PTSD. He suggests: "MIPS may also represent the physical manifestation of an anxiety or depressive disorder, including PTSD. In a significant proportion of individuals with MIPS, there is no adequate psychosocial or biomedical explanation for the symptoms" (p. 199).

The trauma and traumatic memories can be the basis of the pain or serve to exacerbate the pain related to injuries or disease. Beckham, Crawford, et al. (1997) found veterans who had an increase in PTSD re-experiencing symptoms also experienced increased pain levels, pain and disability. The most common source of PTSD is motor vehicle accidents (Blanchard & Hickling, 2003b). According to their research, 15 to 45% of persons in serious motor vehicle accidents may develop PTSD. However, childhood physical and sexual abuse and war are also much too common sources and are significantly correlated with a variety of pain and medical disorders as mentioned above.

There are several models that have been developed to explain the high correlation between PTSD and persistent pain. These include the Mutual Maintenance model (Sharp & Harvey, 2001). Friedman, McEwen, et al. (2003) discuss the relationship of PTSD, allostatic load and medical illness, including pain dis- orders. Other models include shared vulnerability and fear–avoidance (Otis, Keane, & Kerns, 2003) Further, the shared neurological processes of PTSD and persistent pain may exacerbate each other (Asmundson, Coons, et al., 2002; Schnurr, et al., 2003; Friedman, McEwen, et al., 2003; Meagher & Kendall- Tackett, 2003; Schnurr & Green, 2003; Sharp & Harvey, 2001).

Flashbacks and the re-experiencing of symptoms are a common characteristic of PTSD where the person re-experiences all or part of a traumatic memory. Somatosensory flashbacks can result in the re-experiencing of the sensations of the original trauma. Salomons, Osterman, et al. (2004) studied pain flash- backs related to surgery and found significant similarity in the revivification and the original experience In addition, the treatment and reduction of PTSD may result in the reduction of pain (Shipherd, Keyes, et al., 2007). Beckham, Crawford, et al. (1997) reported a significant association of increased pain levels with increased re-experiencing of symptoms.

In this chapter, we focus primarily on dealing with specific traumatic memories that may be related to the experience of persistent pain or triggered during procedures. However, underlying traumatic memories that are not specifically related to the expression of pain can also be resolved by these techniques.

## Case Examples

A young African-American woman being treated for severe recurring rectal pain without resolution was referred to me (JHS). With the use of an affective bridge during light hypnosis she remembered being anally raped with a Coke bottle by several male cousins when she was about 8 years old. She was embarrassed and uncomfortable going into any details about the episode. I explained a version of the movie theater technique to her and how she would not need to talk about any of the details of what happened in order to heal the memory. (While some- times it is valuable for the patient to have someone hear his or her story, accept- ing the patient as a person while acknowledging the trauma of the experience, it is often more comfortable for them to be able to process the memory without having to share the details. This is especially true with memories that involve sexual abuse and degradation.) The total process with this woman took about 45 minutes. Twenty-five years later she reported no recurrence of the pain.

A 37-year-old Caucasian woman had been stabbed multiple times during a rob- bery of the store in which she was working and was still experiencing pain from the area of the wounds as well as anxiety more than a year after the event. With the resolution of the traumatic memories, she no longer experienced the pain and there was a significant reduction in her anxiety levels.

A middle-aged Caucasian woman was experiencing significant pain in her chest area two years after open heart surgery. While she did not have the initial conscious memory of experience, with the use of an affective/kinesthetic bridge she recalled awakening when she was in ice following the surgery. When this memory was resolved, so was the pain.

Sometimes, beliefs anchored to key decisions result in behavior patterns that lead to behavioral patterns that exacerbate existing problems. A middle-aged Caucasian farmer with significant back problems kept reinjuring himself by not restricting his activities. He was referred due to his non-compliance. He held a strong belief that he was not a "real man" (gaining his father's love and acceptance) if he gave into the pain, which would mean he could no longer do much of the physical labor required to run his farm. His key decision memory that was at the basis of his belief was identified and reworked. This resulted in his willingness to comply with the physician's guidelines and still feel like a whole acceptable man.

It is important to consider the possibility of prior trauma when the patient is not responding well to traditional treatment even when the history of related trauma is not obvious. Further, studies suggest a significantly higher history of abuse incidence and PTSD in patients with pelvic pain, IBS and other gastrointestinal problems, fibromyalgia and facial pain. Veterans wounded in combat with a prior history of PTSD report, on average, more significant pain and disability (Aaron, Herrell, et al., 2001; Asmundson, Wright, et al., 2003; Beckham, Crawford, et al., 1997; DeCarvalho, 2004; Howard, 1996; Lampe, Solder, et al., 2000; Longstreth, 1994; Martinez-Lavin, 2001; Namenek, 2006, Roy-Byrne, Smith, et al., 2004; Sherman, 1998).

## Dentistry

As many dentists and oral surgeons are aware, people who have experienced sexual abuse, particularly oral abuse, often avoid dental treatment and can be easily triggered during the procedures. Some patients do not want to discuss their past traumatic experiences and some patients are not consciously aware of their abuse background, especially childhood sexual abuse, and have not figured out their pattern of avoidance (Santos, 1997). It is still helpful to screen patients for any history of oral sexual abuse or trauma.

What is most helpful for patients with trauma histories is having an empathic and understanding dentist who is willing to listen to their concerns. Further, the ability to control how their dental treatment proceeds with a way to stop the procedures eases anxiety. While these are common steps for most patients, they are even more important and may require more detailed and explicit implementation for this population of patients. The use of hypnosis needs to emphasize the patient's control and how the tools provided help the patient have more control over the situation and the experience of the procedure. (See Appendix III at the end of the chapter for a procedural guide.)

## *Memories*

Alfred Adler's Individual Psychology emphasized how early memories served as templates for beliefs and goals as well as other aspects of a person's phenomenological structure. He observed that when an individual made deeper change in therapy, related early memories would change in terms of content, quality or affective intensity. Deep structure therapies focus on modifying early created neuropatterns – which include origin memories, ratification memories, affective reaction, learned stimulus significance, beliefs, decisions and behavioral-response patterns (often considered procedural memories), and are related to key goals such as survival, belonging, mastery, identity. More recent work (Straub, 1995–2002) suggests that these early created neuropatterns are centered in the limbic system, primarily the hippocampus with some immediate survival patterns and learned stimulus significance associated with the amygdala. Further, a visceral response to these patterns often occurs which intensifies the individual's response to these neurobehavioral patterns. Evidence suggests the vagal system may be a primary conduit triggering the visceral response. These neuropatterns are well entrenched and are not easily changed by simply learning that they are not accurate or useful at the prefrontal cortex level. This disconnect between the prefrontal cortex and the limbic system results in the "I know it in my head but not my gut" response.

Various abreaction approaches to traumatic memories that were used in the 1970s, 1980s, and even into the 1990s tended to use a desensitization approach with repeated exposure to the trauma until closure was reached and the intense affective response pattern was unhooked. These abreactive approaches and the outcome restructuring was often not focused and partial resolution or less constructive reframes or restructuring were a result.

In the mid-1970s, Bandler, Grinder, Dilts and others began publishing the results of their work and offering training around it. Their work led to a variety of new ways to think about trauma and memories. They had begun applying modeling tools to what various successful therapists did as opposed to what they said they did. They modeled the work of Virginia Satir, Milton Erickson, Robert Goulding, Fritz Perls and others. Although they created little that was new, they did systematize ideas and approaches from a variety of disciplines. They called their approach Neurolinguistic Programming (NLP), which was an approach to understand how people function and dysfunction.

In NLP the focus is on how individuals develop and maintain internal patterns and strategies, and how therapists can identify and modify patterns and strategies that are limiting, and teach (install) new and more effective patterns and strategies, often using hypnotic techniques. The key to NLP was helping practitioners learn an active, curious approach and apply various modeling tools to better understand their patients' behaviors and patterns in terms of structure, function and context.

As a byproduct of this approach, a variety of tools and techniques were refined or rediscovered and taught. In many ways, what resulted was an integration of hypnosis and cognitive therapy. What many professionals found most useful was a more effective way of directing their curiosity about how people functioned. While most of the tools and techniques were familiar to experienced therapists, some areas that were explored and developed through NLP had very little systematic application in therapy.

Submodalities were one such area. Submodalities are the characteristics of modalities (visual, auditory, proprioceptive, kinesthetic, olfactory, gustatory), such as distance, size, volume, pitch, color, clarity, intensity and so on. Whereas modification of submodalities has been commonly used in imagery work for centuries, Robert Dilts and others began to more systemically explore how people use them as an internal coding system to rapidly convey meaning. In memory work, submodalities can be used both to facilitate the resolution of memories and to provide feedback to identify unresolved issues.

Another area that was refined was the systematic and rapid resolution of trauma and trauma-induced phobias. The visual-kinesthetic (VK) dissociation approach to trauma and the widely used and modified Rapid Phobia Cure (Straub, 1987), often known as the "movie theater technique," were developed. (An effective and powerful version of the movie theater is outlined in Appendix II in this chapter.) Though these approaches drew heavily from the work of Milton Erickson and others, they differed in that they provided a simpler, faster and more targeted application. Over the decades, the authors and others have modified and applied these approaches to help patients more effectively resolve traumatic memories and related affective and belief patterns.

## Resolving Traumatic Memories

It is important to remember that the patient is dealing with a memory, not with the event or the past. The event no longer exists. Only the memory of the event along with the beliefs, understandings and decisions he or she created during and after the event now exist. The brain structures, organizes and stores memories in a variety of ways. Although many memories appear to be accessed through the hippocampus, some intense traumatic memories may be tied to the amygdala. Further, these memories may be more fragmented. Memories and affective beliefs tend to be related to the limbic system and accessed differently from everyday analytical thinking. These thoughts are often labeled "feelings" since they are thoughts with an affective component related to vagal activation.

For key decision memories without major trauma (major trauma occurs when a person perceives that his or her life or physical integrity, or that of another, is or may be threatened), the goal is to help the patient create new, more useful decisions, beliefs and understandings from the event. Sometimes the new understanding is that the event is over and no longer has any significance.

For traumatic memories, the goal usually includes helping the patient bring closure to the memory with as little pain and as much growth as possible in the context of therapy. This includes both facilitating a separation of the memory from the patient and the patient, including parts, from the memory (dissociation from the memory rather than from self or parts) and the restructuring of the patient's limiting beliefs created or reinforced with the trauma. In addition, the development of new, more useful understandings and beliefs is fostered.

Other examples of core belief sets include: *I'm going to die; I am bad; It was my fault; I never show my anger; I must never make Father (men) angry; I am weak; The world is unpredictable and dangerous; Men are dangerous.* These particular beliefs were attached to the memory of a woman reporting esophageal pain and choking. This was related to a memory from when she was 9 years old. Her father had come home drunk and began to fondle her. When she resisted, he choked and brutally raped her. After that, he took his daughter as his mistress.

The most common goals of the approaches discussed here are for the patient to glean useful understandings from the experience, be free of the limiting and detrimental beliefs associated with it, be free from affect and physical sensations connected to it, and to put the memory in the past, coded as something that happened and is over with.

An alternative outcome is to restructure the memory in such a way that new, useful understandings and affect are attached to the memory and the memory is kept active. A third option is to simply strip the memory of affect, intensity and beliefs so that it is more or less erased or is made a neutral memory.

Two overall approaches to resolution are discussed here. One is primarily a submodality approach; the second is a detailed version of the movie theater technique. They both serve to help the patient dissociate from the memory.

Some of the techniques outlined are more effective for overall reframing, some for rapid resolution.

The basic techniques can be modified and combined in a variety of ways depending on the needs of the patient, time limitations, and the memories being processed. For example, when there is single-incident trauma, where memory fragments are separate with little or no meaning attached to them, little or no formal restructuring may be required. Once the memory has been retrieved and put together as a complete narrative experience, the processing will often result in sufficient framing or reframing to achieve the goal. When there is a single-incident trauma such as a car accident, where there are no significant shifts in the patient's phenomenological structure, simply separating the patient from the memory and bringing closure to it using the movie theater technique can be sufficient.

Before working with a patient to resolve a memory, just as with any other intervention, it is important to understand the function of the memory in the patient's life to make sure changes or modifications will be ecologically sound. During the processing of the memory, it is also important to attend to the effect of restructuring. For example, one woman who was referred for treatment experienced severe chest pain. It turned out that this principally occurred when she was around drugs or thinking of using. The pain served to reinforce her decision not to use and in particular not to drive while high (which had been a pattern). As she understood the underlying purpose of the pain, she realized she was not yet certain that she would not use without the help of the pain. The pain was left in place but without the related anxiety and with a new appreciation of its purpose.

The victim identity that is often encouraged in our society provides both primary and often secondary gain. The role of the provider is to lead the patient to more useful understandings and perceptions and away from the belief that she or he is a victim. While the person may have been victimized, he or she did not *become* a victim. Instead, the patient can develop a more positive and useful self-image and often find other ways of achieving the underlying secondary gains or let go of them all together. Related to this can be the problem of the patient feeling sorry for or pitying the younger self rather than having empathy, compassion and respect for him or her. The provider can help the patient focus on the resources, strengths and creativity demonstrated in how he or she coped with the event.

# *Working with the Memory*

Time is often limited in the typical medical practice, but these techniques can be applied in one or two 20–30-minute sessions.

## *The Memory*

Memories have a beginning, middle and an end. The first step after working through ecological issues, establishing a safety or grounding anchor and discussing the procedure with the patient, is getting to the memory. For the purposes of this process, the beginning is defined as 15 minutes before anything bad occurred. The end is defined as 15 minutes after the event was over and the person felt safe, at least for a time. Sometimes the person does not remember what happened before or after and will need to extrapolate and conjecture. This option works fine.

The patient may indicate that the memory is never over because the abuse continued for years and it still goes on in his or her mind. Or the patient may indicate that he or she never felt safe again. The patient must be helped to understand that the work is with the memory of one specific incident and the point being sought is when he or she knew for a time that nothing more was going to happen. It may be after falling asleep that night at home or in the hospital.

Another difficulty at this step is there may be only segments of the memory available, but this may not be obvious currently. In most cases, the missing elements will come into awareness during the process. This is not uncommon when the patient has significant degrees of dissociation and different parts hold different segments of the memory. When this is the case, a request from the patient for just the part is sufficient. Another technique is to have the patient float very high above the memory and look for its missing parts. They are often perceived as parallel timelines.

## *Dissociating from the Memory*

An effective grounding technique for dissociating from the memory is to have the patient float up and out of the memory, leaving all the emotions, sounds, sensations, smells and so on in the memory. The person is asked to take him- or herself out of the situation so that the image is viewed in the memory, as in a video. The patient may have feelings about what is happening down there, but all the emotions associated with the event are to be left with the event. (Feelings about the event are not emotions. They are thoughts with an affective component.) The patient is to float to a point so high above the memory that none of the feelings or sensations from below can reach him or her. Imagery techniques such as being in the gondola of a hot air balloon can be helpful.

The phrase "parts" is jargon for neuropatterns created around beliefs and decisions and that hold the memory or memories of the related belief. Sometimes they are "stuck" (associated in the memory). When this occurs, it makes it difficult for the patient to dissociate from the memory. Bringing the part out of the memory before processing reduces this problem.

Some memories are held by different parts and are accessible only when the part is active. Sometimes different parts hold different portions of the memory, and those parts need to be resolved together or in portions and then brought together for resolution. The goal is for patients to be dissociated from the traumatic memory rather than dissociated from aspects of themselves.

Once the patient is separate from the memory, a beginning and an end need to be established. The patient then floats to a spot high above 15 minutes after the incident was over and the person believed he or she was safe for the time being. Hypnotic language patterns are very helpful even if not absolutely necessary in this process. If the patient is revivifying the memory, an altered state of consciousness is already in place. Consequently, language patterns are critical. Analog marking and repetition of key phrases and directions are valuable. Whatever the patient sees and hears is part of a memory of an event that is over. The patient should be helped to understand that trying to make the memory different at this point will just keep him or her stuck. The patient is instructed not to narrow his or her focus on any particularly gruesome or painful segment because that will too easily lead to a re-association with the memory. Establishing a signal with the patient that will help him or her dissociate from the memory again is necessary.

At this point, particularly with ongoing child abuse, it is valuable to ask if there are any parts of the memory still down in the memory. If there are, the patient is instructed to bring them up with him or her. How close it is brought in depends on the relationship between the person and the part. The part, or parts, is to leave all the qualities – the feeling, sensations, smells and sounds – of the memory down in the memory. It is not uncommon for parts to be identified later as well. If the patient has a great deal of difficulty staying out of the memory, it is likely that one or more parts are still associated in the memory.

## Extracting Useful Understandings from the Memory

Once the patient is stabilized at a spot high above and 15 minutes after the event was over, the patient should be asked what useful learnings or understandings can be gleaned from this objective position before bringing closure to the memory. Some help and direction is often needed.

The therapist helps the patient focus on the self in the memory rather than on what happened or was done. The patient should be encouraged to understand that he or she did the best they possibly could under the circumstances and with the resources available. He or she should be made aware of resources that were used, the limitations that were in place then and the resources that are available now that were not available at the time.

**A few typical themes for restructuring:**

- It happened to you. It was not about you. It was about the perpetrator.

- See how you did the best you could under the circumstances.

- You survived.

- Focus on the younger you (younger may mean 6 months or 60 years), not what *happened* to you.

- Notice what you did to get through this.

- It is over. Are you ever likely to be in that position again?

- Are you still the same person you were then?

- Beating yourself up does not undo a mistake. What constructive actions can you take?

- Be aware of the strength, creativity, determination (or other quality) that was required to get you through this.

The patient must be able to both subjectively and objectively believe these things for effective restructuring to occur. The provider uses a combination of cognitive restructuring and hypnotic techniques to facilitate this change.

The patient may want to blame the younger self for not having the insight, knowledge or skills that are available now: "I should have known!" It is important to lead the patient to fully understand the event as it occurred, including a realistic assessment of the resources, knowledge and perspective of the time. This assessment includes the likely and perceived consequences of behaving differently. A child taught to obey does not usually have the choice to not obey.

The safety and well-being of the patient and those who are close are important. If a woman is raped after walking into a dark parking lot alone at night, it is not her fault. However, it is important that she learn the realities of the world and the need to take extra precaution at times, no matter how unfortunate this reality is. At the same time, if she overgeneralizes and comes to believe that the world is a dangerous place and that she is always vulnerable, this unnecessarily limits her life. A more useful understanding might be that the world is not a dangerous place. However, it has dangers in it and with knowledge and awareness, safety is usually possible. Staying on guard all the time actually promotes an increased sense of vulnerability.

Sometimes, the patient may say, "I was never the same after that." In this case, the person is encouraged to clarify what the sentence really means. If the meaning is limiting, the person is asked about its derivation and then guided to the understanding that most of the changes are a result of what he or she came to believe and that the belief can be controlled. The significant limitation is usually a generalization or selective abstraction. In these situations there will often be a part of the belief from before the shift and another part from after the shift still in the memory. With resolution, it may be useful to integrate these two parts or patterns.

The patient is requested to float to the beginning point identified earlier. From that point, the patient is asked whether there are any other useful understandings, but the possibility that there might not be is acknowledged. A common example is along the lines of how innocent, young or happy he or she was. The patient needs to have extracted all useful understandings and made the appropriate reframes. The process should be continued until therapist and patient are confident. If something important is missed, it will usually result in difficulty in making the submodality shift to black and white and gray (Straub, 2002).

Again, the patient checks for any parts still in the memory. If there are still some, the patient is guided to bring those parts up. (If a part is missed, it will usually result in difficulty making the submodality shift from three dimensional to two dimensional (Straub, 2002). It should be confirmed that the new understandings have been accepted by the parts that were extracted from the memory. Sometimes the restructuring has fully worked with parts that were extracted. However, it is not uncommon that some additional work needs to be done to fully restructure the parts.

One simple technique for restructuring parts is to have the patient focus on the understanding in question and then move the part behind him or her so the part can "see" it the way the patient does now. Eye Movement Desensitization and Reprocessing (EMDR) can facilitate this process (Straub, 2002). The patient must be supported to continue to move through the process of restructuring the parts.

Once the useful learnings and understandings have been extracted – and the limiting ones confronted – and a better appreciation of the younger self has been facilitated, the patient goes to the next step. At this point, there is a choice point.

## Dialoguing

Sometimes, it is useful to have the person float down into the memory after it is over and dialogue with the "younger self." This step is often useful when there is shame or continuing abuse to deal with as a child. This can help attach the knowledge that he or she survived, has a future and is not alone, which further restructures the associated affect and meaning. This can also serve both to build greater acceptance for the younger self and give a more positive end point to the memory.

## Bringing Closure to the Memory

Once the useful understandings are extracted, the key elements have been reframed so that the patient is no longer trying to change what happened, and no longer believes he or she needs to hold on to the active memory, as well as having taken all the parts of self out of the memory, the memory is ready for closure. Occasionally, by this time, the patient spontaneously makes the shift. More often, some additional processes are needed such as the submodality shifts described in Appendix I of this chapter. Ultimately, the memory will no longer trigger an affective response and submodality shifts will occur (or be facilitated) that indicate the change. The memories will seem over, as something that happened in the past. They often seem smaller, more distant, less clear or fainter.

# Appendixes

Over the last two and a half decades, these approaches and techniques have been modified, developed and refined by the authors utilizing information learned in training with and from published materials by Alfred Adler, Milton Erickson and Robert Goulding. Other material is culled from works in Psychosynthesis, Neurolinguistic Programming (NLP), Timeline Therapy (a branch of NLP developed by Tad James and Wyatt Woodsmall), as well as by Bessel Van Der Kolk and many others. Although many of the elements are related to several sources, the work of Milton Erickson, submodality and NLP techniques provided the beginning structure for the movie theater technique. NLP submodality work is from Robert Dilts and others. Graduate training in Psychosynthesis with Betty Bosdell and research in traditional imagery work were significant in the development and refinement of the submodality approach.

# Appendix I: Submodality Memory Processing

Often negative, limiting or mild-to-moderately traumatic memories can be simply and rapidly processed by extracting all useful understandings, reframing the meaning attached to the memory and then modifying the submodality characteristics of the memory.

## The Process

*Step I: Selecting the beginning and end points of the memory*
When a problematic memory has been selected, the patient is asked to identify a point slightly before anything bad, scary or troublesome began to occur in the memory. Then the patient is requested to select a point after he or she knew the event was over and he or she was safe, at least for the time being. Either or both points may need to be extrapolated or created by what the patient believes is likely to have happened. It should be explained that these points will represent the beginning and end of the memory.

*Step II: Dissociating from the memory*
The patient dissociates from the memory, and is asked to float or step out of the memory and look at and listen to the memory from the outside, as though someone had made a three-dimensional movie of it. "Leave the emotions and sensations of your memory in the memory, and listen to the voices and other sounds coming from your memory. Look at it from above or the side, not from over the shoulder of the image of you in the memory." (It is usually easier for people to float above the memory.)

Once fully dissociated from the memory, the patient floats above it (if the patient is not already there) to a point high above after the memory is over (the point identified earlier). The patient must float high enough to not experience any of the sensations or emotions from the memory down below. The patient may have feelings about what is going on in the memory but not from the memory itself. It is important to make sure the patient has not floated up into a dissociated aspect of the memory, but is grounded in the present circumstance.

*Step III: Extracting useful understandings about the event*
When the patient is comfortable with looking at and listening to the memory from a point high above after the memory was over, the question is asked: "From your here-and-now objective perspective, high above after it is all over, what useful understandings can you take from the memory before you put it away?" The patient may need to be guided through the process to help gain new perspective and reframe the meaning attached to aspects of what happened in the memory.

Sometimes, as mentioned earlier, the patient believes that a negative experience must be held onto in order not to repeat it. The simple analogy mentioned earlier can help. "Do you need to remember the pain of touching the hot burner on a stove to remember not to touch it again?"

It is not uncommon for the patient to still want to change the events of the memory and create an alternative ending. Acceptance of the reality that the event is over and will be better resolved by letting it go should be encouraged. It should be explained that keeping it open only interferes with getting on with life and making changes the patient wants.

The patient should be helped to focus on him- or herself in the memory rather than on what happened or was done to him or her. The awareness that the patient did the best he or she could under the circumstances given the knowledge and resources available at the time should be supported. Further, the patient should be clear about the resources that were used then, and limitations should be normalized. The resources the patient has now, which were not available at that time, should be delineated. Extracting all useful understandings and making the appropriate reframes is essential. See "Extracting useful understandings from the memory" for examples of useful reframes and points. Both patient and therapist need to be sure that this has been accomplished.

*Step III: a*
Next the patient is directed to float to a point high above the memory before anything began. From that point, the patient is asked whether there are any other useful understandings, while stressing that there might not be any. The most common one from this point is along the lines of how innocent, young or happy the patient was at the time. Again, the extraction of all useful understandings is important.

*Step III: b*
Sometimes, when the memory is from childhood, it can be useful for the patient to float down next to the "younger self" after it is all over and talk with the

younger one about what happened. This is a time to affirm that the patient is okay, will survive, is not to blame and so on. When the patient first floats next to the younger self, he or she is asked whether the younger self knows who the patient is. If not, have the patient introduce him- or herself. Then the patient is directed to talk to the younger self and provide nurturing, acceptance, understanding, protection, perspective and so on. This "conversation" not only serves to strengthen the restructuring of the parts, it also helps the provider determine whether the patient has fully accepted the new understandings or is still in some way blaming or rejecting a part of him- or herself.

*Step IV: Identifying and restructuring parts associated with the memory*
The next question: "Is there any part of you still in the memory?" If there the answer is yes, the patient is asked to bring up the part or parts. The patient then has the part(s) look through his or her own eyes at the memory, using the understandings the patient now has. This method promotes restructuring of the beliefs and understandings of the part(s) by the patient. The process continues until the part(s) have the new understandings.

Sometimes the patient needs to bring up the parts from the memory earlier. This is especially true when the patient is having trouble staying dissociated from the memory. In that case, it is better to keep the part(s) high above, but not next to the patient, as he or she is identifying the useful learnings. Then the patient is helped to restructure the part(s) in the same way as above.

*Step V: Submodality restructuring of the memory – color*
Once the patient has reframed the memory, he or she is asked to make it black, white and gray. Any part that will not change or needs to be forced indicates some issue has not been dealt with. Whatever still has to be addressed needs to be processed until the whole memory is black, white and gray. If, according to the patient, a part is still stuck in the memory, he or she is guided to take the part out of the memory and to help the part process whatever is needed.

*Step VI: Submodality restructuring of the memory – dimension*
After the color has been taken out, the patient is directed to make it flat, like a series of black-and-white photographs. If a part of the memory will not go flat, it is an indicator that more work needs to be done. In this case, it is more likely to be a part still in the memory.

*Step VII: Checking for sufficient change*
Once the memory is totally flat and black, white and gray, the status is rechecked by asking the patient how he or she feels when thinking about and looking at the memory as an additional check. The feeling will usually be neutral or sometimes positive.

*Step VIII*
The patient is asked whether there are any sights, sounds, emotions, sensations, smells or tastes from the memory that are still held by the patient or by a part. If held by the patient, he or she is instructed to float above the flat memory and empty everything from the memory back into the memory. If held by the part, the patient helps the part(s) empty everything from the memory back into the memory. If problems are encountered, the possibility that there are still unresolved issues must be revisited.

*Step IX: Framing the memory*
The patient then creates a frame around the memory that indicates, "This is something in the past that is over with, and I do not need the memory anymore. It is just a fact representing something that happened in the past."

*Step X: Putting the memory in the past*
The patient is instructed to move the memory into the past, to the location related to the age when the event occurred. Once again, the patient is asked to look at the memory now that it is in the past and notice the feelings he or she has. A typical feeling is that the memory represents something that is over and done with and just a part of the past.

*Step XI: Desensitizing highly sensitized parts, if needed*
When there are parts that are highly sensitized to certain triggers, imagery rehearsal may be beneficial in desensitizing the parts and further strengthening the restructuring. This is done in the same way outlined in the disidentification process after the parts are moved to a safe and comfortable place well behind the patient's physical body.

# Comments

This simple process will work with a wide variety of memories. It is not usually the best one for severe traumatic memories such as rapes, assaults or severe car accidents, especially if they are recent. However, it will often work with severe trauma from the more distant past, if care is taken. The technique can be used for similar repeated incidents over time. If this is the case, the patient is asked to create a representative memory of the repeated incidents. For example, when parents get drunk night after night and become abusive with each other while the child tries various strategies to help, the child may feel helpless, afraid, a failure. Different parts will hold different strategies that were tried. Each part needs to understand that it is over, that the part did the best it could under the circumstances, that it was not in its power to make it better and so on.

The provider needs to be alert to the patient's overt and covert signals and adaptable as far as what is needed in order for the patient to achieve the desired outcomes. Outcomes include disassociation from the memory, including all parts, reframing and restructuring of the beliefs and meanings, and submodality feedback and restructuring of the memory.

# Appendix II: Rapid Traumatic Memory Restructuring and Resolution: The Movie Theater Technique

## Summary of Essential Steps

### Preparing to process the memory
While the more involved restructuring processes previously described are not necessary for the movie theater technique, they often enhance patient changes, especially when dealing with chronic abuse. The previous steps are necessary for the submodality processing technique.

### The steps
1. Establish rapport, identify primary and secondary gains, and conduct an ecology check.

2. Explain the process to the patient.

3. Facilitate relaxation using hypnotic language patterns.

4. Establish safety anchors.

5. Instruct patient to float to a safe place high above 15 minutes after the incident was over. Anchor that state.

6. Have the patient assess the memory from the safe place and extract any parts that are still down in the memory.

7.  Identify useful learnings, understandings, new beliefs and restructure limiting ones

8.  Have the patient float to the 15-minute-before high-above point and repeat the previous two steps.

9.  Have the patient float back to the 15-minute-after high-above point and review the new understandings.

10. Make sure new beliefs and understandings are fully accepted by the patient and all of the patient parts.

11. Have the patient float to the 15-minute-before high-above point.

12. Have the patient imagine a movie theater far below, just above the memory. The patient is looking into the auditorium of the theater.

13. Have the patient look at a recent black-and-white photo of him- or herself being projected on the screen.

14. Have the patient imagine him- or herself at the age he or she is now walking into the auditorium and taking a comfortable seat looking up at the screen.

15. Then have the patient see himself or herself floating out of the self sitting in the auditorium and up into the projection booth.

16. The patient is instructed from this point on to only focus on the "you" in the projection booth; not on the "you" in the auditorium or the movie.

17. Have the patient direct the self in the projection booth to project a still-pause, black-and-white image of the younger self 15 minutes before the incident begins.

18. Have the patient direct the self in the projection booth to, when signaled, run the black-and-white movie to the end, 15 minutes after the incident was over, pause the final image on the screen and signal when it is over.

19. Repeat the instructions that the patient is to stay focused on the self in the projection booth throughout the running of the movie and to signal or stop if he or she starts to go back into the memory.

20. If the patient is ready, have him or her signal the self in the projection booth to begin running the movie.

21. Continue repeating the instructions to the patient in a quiet, background voice every 30 seconds or so: *Stay high above while you keep your focus on the you in the projection booth and the you in the projection booth focuses on the you in the auditorium. Only the you in the auditorium is watching the black-and-white movie of what happened back then.*

22. When the patient indicates the final scene is frozen on the screen, give these instructions: *Not yet, but in a minute, you will float down into the younger you on the screen. Then you will turn everything back into color and play the movie backward very fast, taking only 3 to 5 seconds so everything will be a blur of sight, sounds and feelings. Do you understand? Are you ready? Float down into the younger you. Turn everything back into color. Play it backward now. And then make a swishing sound. Back...back...back. Are you all the way back to before?*

23. When the patient is all the way back, have him or her come back to the here-and-now room and briefly change the subject. Then ask the patient whether the memory seems different in any way. If there is no difference, some piece of the directions were not given or followed correctly. At this point, a new part of the memory may come into consciousness. If it does, it likely has a part in it that will need to be removed and restructured before going on.

24. Unless the memory is totally resolved, have the patient float back up to above 15 minutes before and repeat the process (adding any new segments that might have been identified), indicating the patient can play all parts of the movie he or she stayed out of. Tell the patient to go through the process faster this time.

25. At the end of running it backward, the patient can stay up above and report how the memory seems now. Repeat the process several times, going faster each time, until the memory is resolved. Then have the patient return to the here-and-now room.

26. Talk with the patient about the experience, and review the restructured understandings and beliefs and how the memory seems now. If there are any problems, repeat the related components. Otherwise, the process is over.

27. Check and review during the next session.

# Appendix III: Dental and Oral Surgery

## Setting the Stage Prior to Procedures

1.  Describe the procedure, ask for a summary to check if the patient understands and grasps the essential aspects of the procedure. Normalize the anxiety response with patients diagnosed with PTSD and persistent pain.

2.  Discuss how to self-calm and ground; inquire about how the patient has done this in the past during stressful or challenging situations. If possible, have the patient practice the self-calming techniques prior to the procedure. Suggest a website (see list) for additional support/ideas.

3.  Establish a signal for stopping the procedure.

4.  Discuss imagery rehearsal of the procedure with anxiety reduction and self-calming strategies integrated into the rehearsal.

## Doing the Procedure

1.  Verbalize the step-by-step components of the procedure: "Now I am…Next, I will…You may feel some pressure…"

2.  Give feedback during the procedure: "Yes, you are remembering to slow your breathing…I see you relaxing your…"

3.  If the patient begins to experience a flashback, use the grounding and self-calming approaches discussed prior to the procedure. Use the steps discussed in the section on resolving traumatic memories in the text above.

## Resources for Patients

Common Fears Download Center <http://www.downloads.dentalfearcentral.org/commonfears.html>

# Bibliography and Resources

Aaron, L. A., Herrell, R., Ashton, S., Belcourt, M., Schmaling, K., Goldberg, & Buchwald, D. (2001). Comorbid clinical conditions in chronic fatigue: A co-twin control study. *Journal of General Internal Medicine*, 16(1), 24–31.

Andreski, P., Chilcoat, H., & Breslau, N. (1998). Post-traumatic stress disorder and somatization symptoms: A prospective study. *Psychiatry Research*, 79(2), 131–138.

Asmundson, G. J. G., Coons, M. J., Taylor, S., & Katz, J. (2002). PTSD and the experience of pain: Research and clinical implications of shared vulnerability and mutual maintenance models. *Canadian Journal of Psychiatry*, 47, 930–937.

Asmundson, G. J. G., & Taylor, S. (2006). PTSD and chronic pain: Cognitive-behavioral perspectives and practical implications. In *Psychological Knowledge in Court: PTSD, Pain, and TBI*. New York: Springer Science + Business Media.

Asmundson, G. J. G., Taylor, S., Young, G., Kane, A. W., & Nicholson, K. (2006). *PTSD and Chronic Pain: Cognitive-Behavioral Perspectives and Practical Implications*. New York: Springer Science + Business Media.

Asmundson, G, J. G., Wright, K. D., McCreary, D. R., & Pedlar, D. (2003). Post-traumatic stress disorder symptoms in United Nations peacekeepers: An examination of factor structure in peacekeepers with and without chronic pain. *Cognitive Behaviour Therapy*, 32, 26–37.

Bandler, R, & Grinder, J. (1975). *The Structure of Magic I*. Palo Alto, CA: Science and Behavior Books.

Bandler, R., & Grinder, J. (1975). *Patterns of the Hypnotic Techniques of Milton H. Erickson*. Capitola, CA: Meta Publications.

Bandler, R., & Grinder, J. (1979). *Frogs into Princes: Neuro Linguistic Programming*. Moab, UT: Real People Press.

Bandler, R., Grinder, J., & Satir, V. (1976). *Changing with Families*. Palo Alto, CA: Science and Behavior Books.

Beckham, J. C., Crawford, A. L., Feldman, M. E., Kirby, A. C., Hertzberg, M. A., Davidson, J. R. T., & Moore, S. D. (1997). Chronic posttraumatic stress disorder and chronic pain in Vietnam combat veterans. *Journal of Psychosomatic Research*, 43, 379–389.

Blanchard, E. B., & Hickling, E. J. (2003a). The role of physical injury in the development and maintenance of PTSD among MVA survivors. In *After the Crash: Psychological Assessment and Treatment of Survivors of Motor Vehicle Accidents* (2nd edn). Washington, DC: American Psychological Association.

Blanchard, E. B., & Hickling, E. J. (2003b). What proportion of MVA survivors develop PTSD? In *After the Crash: Psychological Assessment and Treatment of Survivors of Motor Vehicle Accidents* (2nd edn). Washington, DC: American Psychological Association.

DeCarvalho, L. T. (2004). Predictors of posttraumatic stress disorder in chronic low back pain patients. *Dissertation Abstracts International: Section B: The Sciences and Engineering*, 64, 2004, 4030B.

El-Hage, W., Lamy, C., Goupille, P., Gaillard, P., & Camus, V. (2006). Fibromyalgia: A disease of psychic trauma? *Presse Med*, 35(11 Pt. 2), 1683–1689.

Engel, C. C. (2003). Somatization and multiple idiopathic physical symptoms: Relationship to traumatic events and posttraumatic stress disorder. In *Trauma and Health: Physical Health Consequences of Exposure to Extreme Stress*. Washington, DC: American Psychological Association.

Freidenberg, Brian M., Hickling, H. J., Blanchard, E. B., & Malta, L. S. (2006). Posttraumatic stress disorder and whiplash after motor vehicle accidents. In *Psychological Knowledge in Court.* New York: Springer Publishing Co.

Friedman, M. J., McEwen, B. S., Schnurr, P. P., & Green, B. L. (2003). Posttraumatic stress disorder, allostatic load, and medical illness. In *Trauma and Health: Physical Health Consequences of Exposure to Extreme Stress.* Washington, DC: American Psychological Association.

Geisser, M. E., Roth, R. S., Bachman, J. E., & Eckert, T. A. (1996). The relationship between symptoms of post-traumatic stress disorder and pain, affective disturbance and disability among patients with accident and non-accident related pain. *Pain, 66,* 207–214.

Geuze, E., Westenberg, H. G., Jochims, A., de Kloet, C. S, Bohus. M., Vermetten, E., & Schmahl, C. (2007). Altered pain processing in veterans with posttraumatic stress disorder. *Archives of General Psychiatry, 64*(1), 76–85.

Heim, C., Ehlert, U., Hanker, J. P., & Hellhammer, D. H. (1998). Abuse-related posttraumatic stress disorder and alterations of the hypothalamic-pituitary-adrenal axis in women with chronic pelvic pain. *Psychosomatic Medicine, 60,* 309–318.

Howard, F. M. (1996). The role of laparoscopy in the evaluation of chronic pelvic pain: Pitfalls with a negative laparoscopy. *Journal of the American Association of Gynecological Laparoscopy, 4*(1), 85–94.

James, T., & Woodsmall, W. (1988). *Time Line Therapy and the Basis of Personality.* Cupertino, CA: Meta Publications.

Lampe, A., Solder, E., Ennemoser, A., Schubert, C., Rumpold, G., & Sollner, W. (2000). Chronic pelvic pain and previous sexual abuse. *Obstetrics Gynecology, 96*(6), 929–933.

Longstreth, G. F. (1994). Irritable bowel syndrome and chronic pelvic pain. *Obstetrics Gynecology Survey, 49*(7), 505–507.

McLean, S. A., Clauw, D. J., Abelson, J. L., & Liberzon, I. (2005). The development of persistent pain and psychological morbidity after motor vehicle collision: Integrating the potential role of stress response systems into a biopsychosocial model. *Psychosomatic Medicine, 67,* 783–790.

Martinez-Lavin, M. (2001). Is fibromyalgia a generalized reflex sympathetic dystrophy? *Clinical Experimental Rheumatology, 19*(1), 1–3.

Meagher, M. W., & Kendall-Tackett, K. A. (2003). Links between traumatic family violence and chronic pain: Biopsychosocial pathways and treatment implications. In *Health Consequences of Abuse in the Family: A Clinical Guide for Evidence-Based Practice.* Washington, DC: American Psychological Association.

Meltzer-Brody, S., Leserman, J., Zolnoun, D., Steege, J., Green, E., & Teich, A. (2007). Trauma and posttraumatic stress disorder in women with chronic pelvic pain. *Obstetrics and Gynecology, 109*(4), 902–908.

Namenek, T. M. (2006). The psychopathology of functional somatic syndromes: Neurobiology and illness behavior in chronic fatigue syndrome, fibromyalgia, Gulf War illness, irritable bowel, and premenstrual dysphoria. *Families, Systems, & Health, 24,* 103–105.

Otis, J. D., Keane, T. M., & Kerns, R. D. (2003). An examination of the relationship between chronic pain and post-traumatic stress disorder. *Journal of Rehabilitation Research and Development*, 40(5), 397–406.

Otis, J. D., Pincus, D. B., Keane, T. M., Young, G., Kane, A. W., & Nicholson, K. (2006) Comorbid chronic pain and posttraumatic stress disorder across the lifespan: A review of theoretical models. In *Psychological Knowledge in Court: PTSD, Pain, and TBI*. New York: Springer Science + Business Media.

Roy-Byrne, P., Smith, W. R., Goldberg, J., Afari, N., & Buchwald, D. (2004). Post-traumatic stress disorder among patients with chronic pain and chronic fatigue. *Psychological Medicine*, 34, 363–368.

Salomons, T. V., Osterman, J. E., Gagliesel, L, & Katz, J. (2004). Pain flashbacks in posttraumatic stress disorder. *Clinical Journal of Pain*, 20(2), 83–87.

Santos, C. I. (1997). The identification and treatment of adult female survivors of sexual abuse with dental anxiety. *Dissertation Abstracts International Section A: Humanities and Social Sciences*, 58, 0754.

Schnurr, P. P., & Green, B. L. (2003). Understanding relationships among trauma, posttraumatic stress disorder, and health outcomes. In *Trauma and Health: Physical Health Consequences of Exposure to Extreme Stress*. Washington, DC: American Psychological Association.

Sharp, T. J., & Harvey, A. G. (2001). Chronic pain and posttraumatic stress disorder: Mutual maintenance? *Clinical Psychology Review*, 21, 857–877.

Sherman, J. J. (1998). The identification of posttraumatic stress disorder in facial pain patients. *Dissertation Abstracts International: Section B: The Sciences and Engineering*, 59(1), 0427B.

Shipherd, J. C., Keyes, M., Jovanovic, T., Ready, D. J., Baltzell, D., Worley, V., Gordon-Brown, V., Hayslett, C., & Duncan, E. (2007). Veterans seeking treatment for posttraumatic stress disorder: What about comorbid chronic pain? *Journal of Rehabilitation Research and Development*, 44(2), 153–166.

Straub, J. H. (1987). An eclectic counseling approach to the treatment of panics. *Journal of Integrative and Eclectic Psychotherapy*, 4, 433–449.

Straub, J. H. (1995–2002). *An Introductory Manual for Precision Cognitive Therapy*. Columbia, MO: Human Systems Consultants.

Villano, C. L., Rosenblum, A., Magura, S., Fong, C., Cleland, C., & Betzler, T. F. (2007). Prevalence and correlates of posttraumatic stress disorder and chronic severe pain in psychiatric outpatients. *Journal of Rehabilitation Research and Development*, 44(2), 167–178.

Wald, J., Taylor, S., Fedoroff, I. C., & Taylor, S. (2004). The challenge of treating PTSD in the context of chronic pain. In *Advances in the Treatment of Posttraumatic Stress Disorder: Cognitive-Behavioral Perspectives*. New York: Springer Publishing Co.

## Chapter 11

# Treating Pain, Anxiety, and Sleep Disorders in Children and Adolescents

*Leora Kuttner*

## Introduction and Overview

Hypnosis is an ideal therapy for children and teens. It utilizes creativity, play-fulness, and it relies on imagination. Hypnosis is a child-centered process and requires flexibility to ensure a best fit to each child's individuality. The clinician's intent when using hypnosis is to bring about rapid change in behavior, belief and/or feelings, to free a child from dysfunctional patterns, or to relieve the child of pain and distress (Kuttner, 1997; Olness, 1981, 1996; Sugarman, 1996). Hypnotic language, by itself, can enhance a child's coping ability, and increase self-confidence and comfort. However, when combined with the hypnotic trance experience, which bypasses critical reasoning, old habits, and doubt, change can occur more rapidly and effortlessly. In trance, the child's attention is narrowed, focused, and absorbed, allowing perceptions and sensations to be enhanced, modified, or changed. All humans, and particularly children, have the natural capacity to use an internal imaginative process to affect broad physiologic and psychological changes, particularly with respect to pain modulation (Morgan & Hilgard, 1979; Olness, 1996).

However, hypnosis does not suit all children, or all pediatric problems. It is more difficult to use with a low-IQ or brain-damaged child, it is contraindicated with a fragile or psychotic child, and is more challenging with an unmotivated or conduct-disordered child. Although not a panacea for all pediatric or child-hood problems, in 29 years of practice, I've found hypnosis to be immensely helpful for the following pediatric problems:

*   *Anxiety* – separations, being alone at home, dealing with exam or school performances

- *Sleep problems* – falling asleep, returning to sleep, nightmares, night terrors

- *Acute pain* – needles and invasive procedures, dental procedures, emergency situations

- *Recurrent pain* – tension and migraine headaches, abdominal pain

- *Chronic pain* – concussion, arthritic or joint pain, scoliosis and back pain

In this chapter, we examine how hypnosis can be applied as a therapeutic intervention across the wide age range of ages from young children to late teens (3–19 years) and the changes in hypnotic process necessitated by the different developmental stages. We will close with therapeutic recommendations of how to use hypnosis for the common pediatric problems listed above.

# Applications of Hypnosis Across Developmental Stages

## Newborns and Toddlers – The Preverbal Years

Newborns and toddlers experience the world through sensorimotor interaction. Although hypnosis can be used with children under 3 years old, it has a strong somatic focus, and it is not "true" hypnosis (Morgan & Hilgard, 1979; Olness, 1996). At this age a hypnotic trance state is brief in duration and created in a physical, rhythmic, or ritualized way, for example via familiar lullabies, repeated soothing sounds or words, paired with rapid rocking, rhythmic tapping, or soothing pats. This hypnotic mode reinstates the baby's familiar physical comfort and mimics the maternal heartbeat, which is a rapid 60–70 beats a minute. This somatic and auditory experience entrains the baby's distressed respiration and creates a familiar containment to reduce distress and re-establish the baby's equilibrium. This age-old maternal soothing method of rapid rocking and close contact with rhythmic auditory pulse has been passed on for generations, in cultures where babies are carried on their mother's body.

## Preschools – Simple and Immediate Experiences

Known as the *Magic Years* (6), children from 3–6 years are wonderfully and immediately responsive to hypnotic experiences. Once again, this is not the classic adult hypnotic trance. Preschool children have shorter attention spans, are easily distracted, and weave fluidly between fantasy and reality. They also evidence little physical relaxation during an effective hypnotic trance and often move and wriggle without interfering with its benefit. Furthermore, for children less than 6 years old, closing eyes means going to sleep and they don't wish to do that in the middle of an interesting experience. Hypnotic trance with this age group therefore occurs with the child's eyes wide open. As a result of these differences, Morgan and Hilgard (1979) prefer to call under 6-year-old children's hypnotic experiences "imaginary involvement." Despite the different nomenclature, as well as children's short attention span and desire to keep their eyes wide open, preschool children are generally highly hypnotic and experience rapid and significant behavioral, physiological, and emotional changes and retain the therapeutic benefit of the brief intervention (Kuttner, 1991).

The key to hypnotic success with this age group is to engage the young child with a playful focused interactional style. It is advisable to be flexible, allow the child freedom to move around, and create a vivid and absorbing current experience using their familiar experiences and previous successes. Relaxation usually doesn't occur, and at this age children will be reluctant to close their eyes, so it is not effective to insist upon it (Kuttner, 1991). Sometimes, however, a preschool child can be momentarily fascinated and entranced and their eyes become transfixed when sufficiently absorbed in trance. This age group is charming to work with, but does require an active playful relationship in which movement and action can be part of the trance experience. Trances are short, hypnotic suggestions, which need to be simple and direct, and the outcome is surprisingly significant given the short timeframe (Kuttner, 1986, 1998).

## School-age – Mastery and Growing Self-Control

By 7 years and older children engage in the more classic forms of hypnosis. They are willing to close their eyes, and focus their concentration as they go into trance. Relaxation is not as obvious as with adults, but it does occur and is lighter. Children in this stage of development are the most receptive to hypnosis. Morgan and Hilgard's research (1979) determined that between 8–12 years of age children reach their height of hypnotic talent. Given that all hypnosis is self-hypnosis (Olness, 1981, 1996), it is important to inform school-aged children that this is their talent. With practice they'll be able to use self-hypnosis for themselves wherever and whenever needed. Trances can be longer than with preschool-aged children, a little more indirect but not lengthy (5–7 minutes is a good length). It is always more effective to use the child's own experiences, hobbies, or interests to make the experience relevant, attractive, and absorbing. Gathering this information from the child, parent, or nurse and using it in the trance experience improves cooperation and makes hypnosis more successful.

Useful questions include:

*"If you were not here, what would you rather be doing?"*

*"What do you love to do so much that you don't even hear your Mom/Dad call you?"*

*"Where's your favorite place where you can kind of enter another world?"*

*"What helped in the past when you were worrying?"*

*"Would it be okay if the pain didn't bother you? Instead let's go to that favorite place?"*

The information gleaned from their answers should be woven into an absorbing imaginative experience for the child (Kuttner, 1986, 1991; Olness, 1981). Ideomotor inductions are particularly intriguing for school-age children to use and allow for easier transition to home practice (Olness, 1996). The creation of an audiotape further supports the child's self-hypnosis, self-regulation, and practice at home.

## Teenage Years – Independence and Confusion

Akin to adults, teens enter trance more slowly, and enjoy indirect suggestion and metaphor, a slower, calmer pace with time to relax and release tension in order to shift more deeply into trance. They are capable of sustaining the trance for lengthy periods and engage meaningfully with well-chosen personal contexts. Maintaining their dignity and experiencing independence and respect in the hypnotic process is particularly important to teens. Metaphors that support the teen's growing strengths and sense of adequacy and competency will ensure more effective hypnotic outcome.

The questions listed above for school-aged children also apply to teens and can give an entry into actively participating in their therapeutic hypnotic experience. After hypnotic experiences teens often report their own spontaneous elaborations that reveal the degree to which the trance was made personally relevant. This is important to heed and reintegrate within subsequent hypnotic sessions, as it builds legitimacy for the teen's inner world and supports therapeutic change.

Permissive language, the language of invitation rather than authoritative language, is particularly important to use with teens. It empowers them and furthers their willingness to practice at home. The more the teenager can take on responsibility, practice self-hypnosis at home on a regular basis using an individualized audiotape made in the session, the better the teen's outcome and increasing sense of competency. Developing identity and self-worth is one of the primary tasks of the teenage years.

## Parental Presence During Hypnosis

Younger children will feel more secure and trust professionals more readily if accompanied by a parent for the first session. Parental presence in subsequent sessions is determined by the child, parent, and clinician. In my practice with younger children I often continue to invite parents to sit quietly in the room while the child and I do our hypnotic work for subsequent sessions, unless the presenting problem or issues contraindicate this, or the child verbally or non-verbally shows a preference for time alone with me. The benefit is that parents appreciate the process more substantively, and learn about the power of hypnotic language to support and maintain their child's change. In the session parents will spontaneously close their eyes and accompany their child's hypnotic experience, and in so doing, gain more understanding, appreciation, and value for the process. Consequently, parents are more likely to support the child's ongoing hypnotic home practice hypnosis. This is a system-sensitive way to encourage parents to become allies (Gardner, 1974; Mize, 1996).

## Induction – The First Step in the Hypnotic Experience

Induction is the process by which the child is led into experiencing a hypnotic trance (Olness, 1996). The therapeutic process focuses and narrows attention, leading the child into greater attention absorption so that the child enters an altered state of consciousness. Once in a trance, the therapeutic work can occur: providing suggestions, creating dissociation from the pain and anxiety, and instilling posthypnotic suggestions for positive outcome (Gardner, 1974; Kohen & Olness, 1987; Mize, 1996).

A wide variety of induction techniques are available such as visual and auditory imagery, eye-fixation, ideomotor techniques, and simple relaxation (Kuttner, 1991; Mize, 1996; Olness, 1996). Some useful examples for children follow:

## Visual Imagery Induction

*"Imagine your favorite place…I'm not sure exactly where it is, but you know it very, very well…It's a place where you like to be, where you feel comfortable and happy…You may want to close your eyes so you can see it more clearly…take your time so that you can smell the smells, see clearly, feel what it's like there and hear the sounds. When you're here at your favorite place let me know, by wiggling your finger…"*

## Ideomotor Induction

Ideomotor inductions use the child's own movement to help the child induce trance. These types of inductions are particularly useful to promote the notion of gaining control over one's own body, and therefore over the pain, stomach butterflies, or nausea.

> *"Stand with your arms straight out in front of you so that they are about 10 inches apart. There's a powerful magnet pulling your arms together…Just let it happen… allow your arms to come together…watch it happen. When they touch together, it's a signal to let all the tightness and tension out of your body, to let go…If you wish, close your eyes and take a deep satisfying breath, immediately becoming more comfortable…Take another deep breath in…As you let your breath out notice how and where your body is beginning to feel easier, looser, and more comfortable…"*

## Relaxation

As part of hypnosis, relaxation is generally only utilized with children older than 6 years. It is not a critical component of a child's trance, and may be impossible for the child in acute pain (Kuttner, 1988, 1991; White & Epston, 1990). However, for the child in ongoing or recurring pain, or with a chronic illness, learning how to relax has long-term benefits. In learning the relaxation process (general or progressive relaxation, or site-specific relaxation), the child retrains and eases muscle rigidity and tension, and gains a sense of well-being.

Here is an example: In a pre- or postoperative situation with a young child for whom sleep is desirable, but where the direct suggestion of sleep would meet with resistance, the child's transitional object of his Teddy Bear is used as indirect suggestion for sleep:

> *"What does your bear do when he goes to sleep? You hold him how he likes to be held. Let him get even more comfortable. Pat him…Is he getting sleepy? Let his head get comfortable…Pat his tummy nicely…Let his arms get sleepy and comfortable. Now the bear is feeling sleepy all over…so cozy…so comfortable…so easy…so good to go into a soft safe sleep…"*

## Hypnotic Suggestions – Catalyst for Therapeutic Change

Hypnotic suggestions are given to generate changes in physiology, behavior, and emotions. Suggestions can be directly stated as in, "You'll feel even more comfortable as your eyes close and your breath releases out," or they can be indirectly stated. With children and teens this means using a surrogate via a favorite story, animal, or toy: "As the teddy's head flops, notice how he is becoming happier and happier...he knows that it's going to be OK and his tummy will feel happy too."

In pediatrics, hypnotic suggestions will often promote ego-strengthening, an improved sense of self-worth, courage, and a willingness to take on new behaviors or a more positive attitude to others and upcoming change. The suggestions can be simply stated or embedded within a story and have a surprising impact in facilitating change. In dealing with anxiety or pain, suggestions given sometimes promote distancing or dissociation from the physical and psychological distress. Techniques can range from distraction into a favorite place to suggestions for direct hypnoanalgesia such as the "Magic Glove" or the "Pain Switch" (Kuttner, 1986). Distancing suggestions move the pain away from the child or transfer the pain to another part of the body where it can be more easily released. Suggestions for this distanciation or dissociation can be placed within a metaphor or familiar story (Kuttner, 1998). In the section that follows hypnosis is applied as therapy to some common pediatric problems.

# Common Pediatric Problems

## A. Anxiety and Sleep

Anxiety problems in their many different manifestations are very common in childhood and can present at home or at school. One common presentation is sleep disruption. Both anxiety and sleep problems are wonderfully amenable and responsive to hypnotic intervention (Kuttner, 1997; Olness, 1981, 1996). In taking a history it is important to note the details of the problem presentation. These must be integrated into the hypnotic experience to join the child and facilitate positive change.

### Common Sleep Problems

Children or teens can present with a range of sleep problems: difficulty falling asleep, trouble staying in bed, fear of intruders, being oversensitive to sounds in the house, or attempting to control their parents' movements and presence at night in order to avoid falling asleep. Sometimes this can take the form of waking up during the night, crawling into their parents' bed, or waking a parent for comfort. Nightmares are also a common part of childhood. Less common and more difficult to treat are night terrors.

## Common Anxiety Problems

Anxiety can present somatically, socially, or emotionally. Somatically, children can express anxiety with complaints about nausea, constraints or restraints on eating, fear of throwing up, tightness in the throat or "butterflies." Emotional or social anxiety presents with children becoming clingy with parents, being reluctant to spend time with a new playmate, or refusing to go to school. These are not pathological but common developmental processes, and very amenable to hypnotic suggestion, such as for anxiety reduction, increase in comfort, and growing competency in negotiating this change.

It is helpful to conceptualize children's anxiety problems as a function of *an over-active imagination* (Kohen & Olness, 1987; Kuttner, 1988; Olness, 1996). This talent to create and believe fanciful scenarios, which, in this case, is about catastrophe, should be explained to the child. These scenarios then create feelings of being overwhelmed, helpless, or incompetent – a talent that works against the child's well-being. Invite the child to use imagination to make life different in interesting and surprising ways. This therapeutic dialogue becomes the preparatory material for trance work and sets the stage for entering a trance. "Why not use your brain's talent to imagine and to help you!"

Here are a number of favorite hypnotic metaphors that work well with anxiety problems. What these metaphors have in common is the shift in the power differential between competency and anxiety so that anxiety no longer has the heightened power. For children the experience of being able to cope and feel competent is a powerful anxiolytic. Since anxiety also plays into sleep dysfunction, the following also covers anxieties at bedtime that interfere with the transition into sleep.

## Useful Hypnotic Suggestions and Metaphors for Anxiety and Sleep

1.  For school-aged children, a useful metaphor is anxiety as being like a primitive fungus that grows in dark, dank environments, but when you expose it to the light it begins to shrink, can't grow, and dries up. The more you keep it to yourself, closed in and feed it dark fears, the more it grows and increases, like mushrooms in the forest.

    *"Let's put it in the sunlight, expose it and find out where it likes to hang out, what it attaches to…and what thoughts, pictures, and fears allow it to grow and stop you from feeling and knowing the truth that you are truly safe…"*

    The clinician and child can explore where and when the anxiety appears and how to "open things so that the light shrivels it up." This is a powerful metaphor for change, discussion, and disclosure for school-age children who are natural little scientists, and for teens who understand inhibition. This should be explored before the hypnotic trance to enable the child or teen to engage with understanding this process. Through this discussion the clinician gains a deeper appreciation of the shape, dimension, and scope of anxiety in order to create a hypnotic trance that is a "best fit" to experience a corrective emotional experience. Experiencing both anxiety that is disempowered and a healthy relationship to the previously feared situation needs to occur within the trance experience.

2.  For a younger or school-aged child, a useful process is to objectify the anxiety as a *"creep – clearly not a true friend, but something that isn't invited into your heart, head, or home but creeps or slinks in uninvited and bothers you."* In this example we're borrowing from White and Epston (1990) and the Deconstructionist or Narrative school of psychotherapy, where the problem is deconstructed and dissociated from the self, and in the process the self is empowered. This metaphoric narrative is carried into the hypnotic trance, in which the child can experience, for example, closing the door on *the creep* so that she sets a clear limit on the creepy anxiety and redefines her strength; or counters *"the creep's words of worry"* with newfound *"words of courage and competence."* These can become posthypnotic power phrases that reinstate coping thoughts and behavior well beyond the hypnotic trance and facilitate generalization of new coping skills.

3.  Using the letter "S" to create a new playful reality for the physiological experience of sleep.

    *Curling up into an "S" into your bed…now feel the sweet soft satisfying secure sensation of settling into an "S" position for "S" ssssssleep. Sinking safely into your sheets and softly sounding your breath as stillness seeps into your body and settles you so still and safely that you sink into a sweet soft sleep…*

    This is particularly effective for problems in falling asleep when the child is restless, and caught up in thoughts or anxieties of the day. Here the hypnotic focus is on the child's breath and somatic changes noted in a sibilant soothing manner, which creates a strong sense of security at home, comfort in bed, and trust in her body to allow sleep to occur.

4.  The experience of night terrors is a relatively uncommon problem of childhood. However, those who have it, often have amnesia for the night terror episodes, most of which occur nightly at the same time each night, often after 90 minutes of sleep. These terror episodes are extremely distressing and disruptive for the family. Where night terrors are experienced, the age range is usually 3–7 years. For these children, it is helpful to use a ritualized

active and protective ceremony set to a favorite song. This song is sung by the parents and becomes a hypnotic trance (Kuttner, 1988, 1991). Repeated as the child is in bed as part of the bedtime routine, this hypnotic singing ritual, with the parent as the chief protector, needs to be systematically experienced every night for at least five weeks for significant change in the presentation of the night terrors to occur. This problem is not conducive to a quick fix because of the years of habituation and amnesia that often accompany night terrors. Often these children have experienced years of night terrors before they finally come for treatment, since the standard response is that they'll grow out of it. The "trauma" can be so deeply set in the unconscious that it is only months into the regular practice that substantive change is noticed in the night terror presentation and in the energy and mood of the affected child. This hypnotic ritual is a powerful corrective experience. The metaphor of the protective shield works effectively and can be added to the hypnotic singing ritual. Some progress is often evident within a few weeks but complete resolution can take a few months.

# B. Pain Problems: Acute, Recurrent and Chronic

- Acute pain: needle/invasive procedures, dental procedures

- Recurrent pain: tension and migraine headaches, abdominal pain

- Chronic pain: concussion, arthritic/joint pain, scoliosis pain

## Hypnosis for Pain

Hypnosis, over the last 25 years, has been effectively used and creatively adapted to help children through acute painful experiences in a range of pediatric settings: in the emergency room (White & Epston, 1990), through invasive medical procedures associated with cancer, like bone marrow aspirations and lumbar punctures (Ellis & Spanos, 1944; Genius, 1995; Kellerman, Zeltzer, Ellenberg, & Dash, 1983; Kuttner, 1989; Kuttner, Bowman, & Teasdale, 1988; Liossi & Hatira, 1999; Smith, Barabasz, & Barabasz, 1996; Zeltzer & LeBaron, 1982) and with postoperative pain (Lambert, 1996; Rapkin, Straubing, & Holroyd, 1991). In chronic and persistent conditions it has been successfully used for children suffering with sickle cell disease (Dinges, Whitehouse, et al., 1997; Zeltzer, Dash, & Holland, 1979), burns (Berstein, 1963; Bonham, 1996; Ewin, 1986; Patterson, Questad, & Boltwood, 1987; van der Does, van Dyck, & Spijker, 1988), and tension and migraine headaches (Olness, MacDonald, & Uden, 1987; Smith & Womack, 1987). Research reviews consistently conclude that hypnosis helps children in pain (Chaves, 1994; Tan & Leucht, 1997; Vessey & Carlson, 1996) and should be thought of as an essential component of any comprehensive approach to pain management for children.

Hypnosis can be easily integrated into medical and nursing interventions to reduce distress, relieve pain, and improve outcome. The hypnotic experience with direct or indirect suggestions can enhance coping, heighten the child's sense of safety, comfort, self-esteem and control, and often reduce the need for pain medication. Indeed, hypnosis is a uniquely valuable tool for managing pain (Barber & Adrian, 1982; Hilgard & Hilgard, 1994). As Barber and Adrian (1982) have stated:

> *No other psychological tool that I know of is so efficacious in creating comfort out of discomfort with none of the adverse side effects associated with medical treatments of comparable efficacy.*

Children, particularly those in pain, do not require lengthy inductions, as they are often already in a heightened state of awareness and as such are highly suggestible (Kuttner, 1989). Often only seconds of time are required with a practiced clinician to achieve desired change (Barber, 1977). Hypnosis should be common in the armamentarium of pediatric professionals, introduced early in the treatment process, and certainly not be reserved as a therapy of last resort when the child is tired, sore, and in despair.

The process of hypnosis suits the involuntary nature of pain. Suggestions for pain relief can be highly effective and bypass the child's conscious effort. The ultimate form of hypnosis is *self-hypnosis*, which is ideal for recurring pain and gives control directly to the child to engage in this process whenever and wherever pain occurs. In the management of many chronic habit problems or pain conditions, the child's self-management is crucial to long-term success, underlining the requirement that hypnosis be taught early on, preferably at time of diagnosis, as it empowers the child's coping capacity during the vicissitudes of therapy. The ability to modulate pain and increase comfort furthers the child's sense of independence and self-sufficiency, reducing feelings of helplessness and depression. It often decreases reliance on medication and hospital staff (Tan & Leucht, 1997). In short, hypnosis can be adapted to suit the child with chronic and recurring pain as well as the child with acute pain.

## Children in Acute Pain

### The Emergency Room

Hypnosis has a special role in the emergency room, as children often arrive in pain and in a state of heightened awareness, which is a clear prerequisite for effective hypnotic trance. The hectic atmosphere of the ER, the sudden dislocation from the familiar, parents' anxiety, and the child's fear of the unknown all contribute to the child's anxiety, narrowed focus, and intensified concentration – and its potential for hypnotic suggestion.

There is often a prejudice among ER staff that there is not enough time to address these issues, and that *the child must be held down to be sutured*, but the skillful and incisive use of pediatric hypnosis can be especially effective – particularly for children of 3 or 4 years old. There are few things as reassuring as a medical professional arriving on the scene to teach the child how to help him- or herself through a frightening situation, using breathing, relaxation, and imagination. Hypnosis immediately satisfies the child's need for a sense of control, the parents' need to feel trust in ER staff, and ER staff's need to convince the family that suturing a wound can be painless.

Hypnosis changes the child's focus from needles, respirators, medications, and procedures, to favorite place or favorite activity that soothes and provides comfort. Within minutes the tenor of the room changes from fearful to more manageable (Ellis & Spanos, 1944; Kellerman, Zeltzer, Ellenberg, & Dash, 1983; Kuttner, 1986, 1989, 1991, 1998; Kuttner, Bowman, & Teasdale, 1988; Zeltzer & LeBaron, 1982). Hypnotic analgesia should be used routinely as a pain management method in itself or adjunctive to analgesics in any number of medical settings. The *Pain Switch* and the *Magic Glove* are the two useful hypnotic techniques for acute, recurring, and chronic pain with children:

## *Hypnoanalgesia – The Pain Switch*

This technique is very helpful for children with recurring or ongoing chronic pain. Children with migraines or tension headaches become quite practiced at using the Pain Switch and reliance on medication is notably reduced (Olness, MacDonald, & Uden, 1987).

The idea that the brain controls the body needs to be explained in developmentally appropriate language to the child or teenager.

> *"The nerves send their pain message directly to the brain where it is interpreted and made sense of. The brain then immediately sends these messages back to the body. By focusing attention on the switches that control the incoming pain messages and learning to turn them down, our body then receives a dimmer pain message – the gates close down and we feel less pain. Now concentrate, close your eyes, go into the center of your brain where the switches are (the thalamus for a teen), find the switch in your brain that connects to the part of your body that is hurting…nod your head when you've found it…notice what color it is and type of switch and now take a big deep full breath and as you breathe out turn your pain*

*switch down...notch by notch...at each notch you'll notice slightly less pain...its very interesting...continue going as far down as possible so you'll become more and more comfortable..."*

## Hypnoanalgesia – The Magic Glove

This simple and highly effective hypnotic method takes approximately three minutes and its impact is dramatic in diminishing a child's pain and anxiety (Kuttner, 1986, 1998). Children between the ages of 3–10 years are particularly responsive.

### Procedure

A "Magic Glove" is placed on the selected hand with firm repeated strokes from the tips of the hand to above the wrist, ensuring that each finger is placed in the glove. How the Magic Glove is going on is explained, all the while protecting the hand so that the child *"knows what is happening, but won't be bothered by the procedure."* It should be added that the child may feel some pressure but once again, won't be bothered by it, because the Magic Glove is on and it protects the hand. The other hand is tested for full sensation by poking it with a pencil tip and comparing the sensation rated on a scale of 10 to a similar poke on the gloved hand. The difference should be noted and the child's sensory gains confirmed. With the Magic Glove on, the procedure can proceed with minimal concern and with more confidence. Once the procedure, which is most commonly an IV, is complete it is important to remove the Glove and ensure that sensation is returned to the hand and that there is no longer any sensation difference.

For both hypnoanalgesic procedures, the goal isn't the removal of pain but the diminution of pain and the subsequent feeling of increased control over the pain. As the child becomes more absorbed, the clinician elaborates on the downward modulation for the pain, changing sensations, increasing control and other details as the switch is turned down. The criterion for success is that the child feels a significant difference. For the Magic Glove, the difference is between the "switched-off" area and a complementary unaffected area; for the Pain Switch, the criterion is the difference between pain score before and after the switch was turned down as far as it could go. The Pain Switch technique is particularly useful for children with chronic or recurrent pain problems.

## Children with Chronic, Recurrent Pain

Most children are highly motivated to get rid of pain. This is particularly true for the child with a chronic illness. Hypnosis can play an important part in conjunction with other therapies to empower the child in chronic or recurrent pain, and diminishing the grip of familiar pain that limits the child's daily life. Hypnosis has been effective, for example, in the treatment and management of rheumatoid arthritis, Crohn's disease, and juvenile migraine and tension head-aches (Olness, MacDonald & Uden, 1987; Smith & Womack, 1987). Developing self-coping skills and greater self-reliance on one's ability to manage, under-stand, and modulate chronic pain helps prevent the onset of depression and dysfunction in children with ongoing and recurring or chronic pain syndromes. Self-management is essential for their armamentarium.

*Cautions*

For the children or teens skilled in hypnotic pain control accustomed to dealing with ongoing or severe chronic pain, there is the risk of under-diagnosis and under-treatment of their pain. In the pediatric medical setting, pain has great signal value as a guide to both diagnosis and treatment. The best assessment remains the child's self-report and, in the case of children with chronic illness, this means paying closer attention and asking and assessing with more detail. Teens and children need to remember that covering up important symptoms with hypnosis can mislead assessments. Headaches can indicate tumors, and stomach aches can indicate Crohn's disease or ulcerative colitis. It is impor-tant that diagnostic information from the child's pain be thoroughly evaluated before the therapeutic use of hypnosis is begun.

# Conclusion

Hypnosis is highly rewarding to use with children. It capitalizes on the child's developmental needs and their prolific imaginations as the agents of change (Gardner, 1974; Kohen & Olness, 1987; Kuttner, 1986, 1988, 1991, 1997, 1998; Mize, 1996; Olness, 1981, 1996; Sugarman, 1996). For a successful outcome, the clinician needs to enter the child's world cognitively, emotionally, and imagi-natively. This experience can be creative and enjoyable for both the clinician and the child. Cognitively, children prior to the teen years are concrete thinkers whose imaginations thrive on favorite activities, themes, and places. They want to believe that their "brain switches can turn off pain" or that discomfort will lessen as they walk through "Candy Land." Hypnosis provides them with the process to create this altered reality and relief. For teens, hypnosis is a means for greater self-control and management.

Children and teens facing distressing or painful experiences seek adults they can trust to help them maintain autonomy, control, and even mastery in the face of challenging circumstances. When children discover that an unpleas-ant, worrisome, or painful experience improves when they use their hypnotic imaginations, the feeling of mastery is exhilarating. The only limits to the ways that hypnosis can be utilized to reduce pain are the limits of the clinician's creativity.

# References

Barber, J. (1977). Rapid induction analgesia: A clinical report. *Am J Clin Hypn*, 19: 138–147.

Barber, J. & Adrian, C. (1982). *Psychological Approaches to the Management of Pain*. New York: Brunner/Mazel.

Berstein, N. R. (1963). Management of burned children with the aid of hypnosis. *J Child Psych Psych*, 4: 93.

Bonham, A. (1996). Procedural pain in children with burns. Part 2: Nursing management of children in pain. *Int J Trauma Nurs*, 2(3): 74–77.

Chaves, J. F. (1994). Recent advances in the application of hypnosis to pain management. *Am J Clin Hypn*, 37(2): 117–129.

Dinges, D. F., Whitehouse, W. G., Orne, E. C., Bloom, P. B., Carlin, M. M., Bauer, N. K., Gillen, K. A., Shapiro, B. S. Ohene-Fempong, K., Dampier, C., & Orne, M. T. (1997). Self-hypnosis training as an adjunctive treatment in the management of pain associated with sickle cell diseases, *Int J Clin Exp Hypn*, XLV(4): 417–432.

Does, A.J.W. van der, Van Dyck, R., & Spijker, R. E. (1988). Hypnosis and pain in patients with severe burns: A pilot study. *Burns*, 14(5): 399–404.

Ellis, J. A. & Spanos, N. P. (1944). Cognitive-behavioral interventions for children's distress during bone marrow aspirations and lumbar punctures: A critical review. *J Pain Sympt Manage*, 9(2): 96–108.

Ewin, D. M. (1986). Emergency room hypnosis for the burned patient. *Am J Clin Hypn*, 29: 7–12.

Fraiberg, S. H. (1959). *The Magic Years*. New York: Scribner's

Gardner, G. G. (1974). Parents: Obstacles or allies in child hypnotherapy? *Am J Clin Hypn*, 17: 44–49.

Genius, M. L. (1995). The use of hypnosis in helping cancer patients control anxiety, pain, and emesis: A review of recent empirical studies. *Am J Clin Hypn*, 37(4): 316–325.

Hilgard, E. R. & Hilgard J. R.(1994). *Hypnosis in the Relief of Pain*. New York: Brunner/Mazel.

Kellerman, J., Zeltzer, L., Ellenberg, L., & Dash, J. (1983). Adolescents with cancer: Hypnosis for the reduction of the acute pain and anxiety associated with medical procedures. *J Adol Health Care*, 4(2): 85–90.

Kohen, D. P. (1986). Applications of relaxation/mental imagery (self-hypnosis) in pediatric emergencies. *Int J Clin Exp Hyp*, XXXIV: 283–294.

Kohen, D. P. & Olness, K. (1987). Child hypnotherapy: Uses of therapeutic communication and self-regulation for common pediatric situations. *Pediatr Basics*, April: 1–10.

Kuttner, L. (1986). *No Fears, No Tears: Children with Cancer Coping with Pain.* Boston: Fanlight Productions.

Kuttner, L. (1988). Favorite stories: A hynotic pain-reduction technique for children in acute pain. *Am J Clin Hyp*, 30(4): 289–295.

Kuttner, L. (1989). Management of young children's acute pain and anxiety during invasive medical procedures. *Pediatrician*, 16: 39–44.

Kuttner, L. (1991). Helpful strategies in working with pre-school children in pediatric practice. *Pediatr Annals*, 20(3), March: 120–127.

Kuttner, L. (1997). Mind–body methods of pain management. In: *Pain Management in Children. Child and Adolescent Psychiatric Clinics of North America*, 6(4): 783–796.

Kuttner, L. (1998). *No Fears, No Tears – 13 Years Later.* 46 minute videotape. Boston: Fanlight Productions.

Kuttner, L, Bowman, M., & Teasdale, M. (1988). Psychological treatment of distress, pain and anxiety for young children with cancer. *J. Dev Behav Pediatr*, 9(6): 374–381.

Lambert, S. A. (1996). The effects of hypnosis/guided imagery on the postoperative course of children. *Dev Behav Ped*, 17(5): 307–310.

Liossi, C. & Hatira, P. (1999). Clinical hypnosis versus cognitive behavioural training for pain management with pediatric cancer patients undergoing bone marrow aspirations. *Int J Clini Exp Hypn*, 47(2): 104–116.

Mize, W. L. (1996). Clinical training in self-regulation and practical pediatric hypnosis: What pediatricians want pediatricians to know. *Dev Behav Pediatr*, 17(5): 317–322.

Morgan, A. H. & Hilgard J. R. (1979). The Stanford hypnotic scale for children. *Am J Clin Hyp*, 21: 78–85.

Olness, K. (1981). Hypnosis in pediatric practice. *Cur Prob Pediatr*, 12: 1–47.

Olness, K. (1996). *Hypnosis and Hypnotherapy with Children.* New York: Guilford Press.

Olness, K., MacDonald, J., & Uden, D. (1987). Prospective study comparing propanolol, placebo and hypnosis in management of juvenile migraine. *Pediatr*, 79(4): 593–597.

Patterson, D. R., Questad, K. A., & Boltwood, M. D. (1987). Hypnotherapy as a treatment for pain in patients with burns: Research and clinical considerations. *J Burn Care Rehab*, 8(4): 263–268.

Rapkin, D. A., Straubing M., & Holroyd, J. C. (1991). Guided imagery, hypnosis and recovery from head and neck cancer surgery: An exploratory study. *Int J Clin Exp Hypn*, 39: 215–226.

Smith, J. T., Barabasz, A., & Barabasz, M. (1996). Comparison of hypnosis and distraction in severely ill children undergoing painful medical procedures. *J. Counsel Psych*, 43(2): 187–195.

Smith, M. S. & Womack, W. M. (1987). Stress management techniques in childhood and adolescence. *Clin Pediatr*, 26(11): 581–585.

Sugarman, L. I. (1996). Hypnosis in a primary care practice: Developing skills or the "new morbidities." *J Dev Behav Pediatr*, 17(5): 300–305.

Tan, S. Y. & Leucht, C. A. (1997). Cognitive-behavioural therapy for clinical pain control: A 15-year update and its relationship to hypnosis. *Int J Clin Exp Hypn*, 45(4): 396–416.

Vessey, J. A. & Carlson, K. L. (1996). Nonpharmacological interventions to use with children in pain. *Issues Comp Pediatr Nurs*, 19(3): 169–182.

White M. & Epston, D. (1990). *Narrative Means to Therapeutic Ends*. New York: W.W. Norton.

Zeltzer, L., Dash, J., & Holland, J. P. (1979). Hypnotically induced pain control in sickle cell anemia. *Pediatrics*, 64: 533–536.

Zeltzer, L. & LeBaron, S. (1982). Hypnotic and non-hypnotic techniques for the reduction of pain and anxiety during painful procedures in children and adolescents with cancer. *Behav Pediatr*, 101(6): 1032–1035.

## Chapter 12

# Evidence-Based Efficacious Hypnosis for Obstetrics, Labor and Delivery, and Preterm Labor

*Donald C. Brown*

The most important five minutes of our lives is the first five minutes after birth. How quickly we adapt to extrauterine life often determines how quick we are the rest of our lives. We are missing a tremendous opportunity by not making hypnosis available to all our obstetric patients. They and their newborn infants have so much to gain, so little to lose (Bobart & Brown, 2002).

## Empirical and Theoretical Rationale for the Use of Hypnosis in Obstetrics

Benefits resulting from the use of hypnosis in obstetrics:

1. Hypnosis has been found to decrease fear, tension, and pain before and during labor. A review found hypnosis was reported consistently as eliminating or greatly reducing the experienced pain of childbirth, with an effectiveness ranging from 35–90%, and a median of 50% (Hoffman & Kipenhaur, 1969).

2. Hypnosis significantly increases the ease and speed of labor (Gross & Posner, 1963; Flowers et al., 1960). When used for anesthesia, analgesia, or sedation in labor and delivery, hypnosis is completely harmless (Weinberg, 1963).

3. Hypnosis allows control of painful uterine contractions (Gross & Posner, 1963; Weinberg, 1963; Hilgard & Hilgard, 1975).

4. Hypnosis reduces the need for medication during delivery (Gross & Posner, 1963; Weinberg, 1963; Moya & Jones, 1982).

5.  Hypnosis reduces postpartum insomnia, headache, and breast discomfort. It fosters speedier recovery following delivery (Gross & Posner, 1963; Weinberg, 1963; Hilgard & Hilgard, 1975; Moya & Jones, 1982).

6.  Hypnosis allows the mother to experience the delivery, primarily as a fulfilled feeling of accomplishment, August 1960).

The use of hypnotic techniques in obstetrics to control pain goes back more than a century (Werner, Schauble, & Knudson, 1982). The key aspect of the use of hypnotherapy in the birth process is the involvement of the patient before the labor process begins, so that she can assist the physician in the labor and delivery (Oster, 1994).

Hypnosis use spans the entire duration of pregnancy, from control of early nausea and vomiting through prevention and control of postpartum depression and anxiety. Reducing the caesarean section rate, controlling elevated blood pressure and hyperemesis, and preventing prematurity are but a few of the valuable effects hypnosis can have on pregnancy. It is important to remember that hypnosis represents but one of the obstetrician's tools. When used in conjunction with other more traditional methods, hypnosis allows obstetricians to best serve their patients (Goldman, 1992). In 1939, Delee wrote, "The only anesthetic that is without danger is hypnotism."

Santiago Roig-Garcia (1961) coined the term "Hypnoreflexogenous method" in which he combined the concept of conditioned reflex with hypnosis and its application to obstetrics. He maintained that suggestion is the simplest and most typical basis of the conditioned reflex in human beings. He accomplished wakefulness without pain in delivery exclusively through conditioning of reflexes based upon previous verbal suggestions given under deep hypnosis.

During the training session the patients are taught alternative ways to produce hypno-analgesia and anesthesia. First, a suggestion is given that if at any time during labor or delivery the patient experiences a contraction that creates significant discomfort, she can automatically lapse into the deepest hypnotic state that she can attain, remain in it as long as the contraction lasts and when the contraction is over she will be completely comfortable again. In a case of extended and fatiguing labor, she may choose to remain in the hypnotic state through several contractions or even through the rest of labor and delivery (Werner, 1959).

Second, patients are taught active imagery techniques whereby they can control and maintain a satisfying depth of hypnosis any time they choose during the prenatal, labor and delivery, or postnatal period. The emphasis throughout the training is that we are not training the patients to undergo surgery, but rather to perform a normal physiological act. We emphasize that this technique prepares the patient for delivery and does not require that she be in a hypnotic state during childbirth.

The primary benefits of using hypnosis with obstetric patients, as noted by Kroger (1977), include: (a) reduction of chemo-analgesia, with the reduction of undesirable postoperative effects due to medication for mother, fetus, and subsequently, the child; (b) reduction of fear, tension, and pain before and during labor, with consequent rise in pain threshold; (c) control of painful uterine contraction; (d) decreased shock and speedier recovery following delivery; (e) greater resistance to fatigue, thus minimizing maternal exhaustion; and (f) allowing mothers to experience the delivery, primarily the fulfilled feeling of accomplishment.

Hypnotic suggestions can lead to a smoother convalescence and shorter hospital stay (Erickson, 1994) and hypnotically trained patients rarely experience postpartum depression (Goldman, 1992). In addition, hypnosis in the use of labor and delivery training can reduce cesarean section rate, control elevated blood pressure, and reduce likelihood of premature birth (Martin, 1987; Knudson, 1984). Making pregnancy safer and more rewarding reduces the stress for both the patient and the physician, and this in turn reduces the risk of malpractice litigation (Goldman, 1992).

The objective of Bobart and Brown's (2002) study was to determine if there was a significant difference in Apgar scores of babies born to mothers who received hypnotic childbirth training compared with matched controls who delivered the same day without hypnosis training. Thirty-six individuals were in each group, and each delivered one baby. The hypnosis group infants had significantly better Apgar scores than the non-hypnosis newborns. Thirty-five of the control patients (97%) received regional anesthesia for delivery compared to 38% (14/36) women in the hypnosis group. Only 5.5% of the hypnosis group required analgesia compared to 75% of the control group who required pre-medication. Hypnosis was successful as the sole anesthetic in 61% of deliveries, while only 2.7% of the control group did not require any anesthetic or premedication. The hypnosis group also had a significantly shorter hospital stay (4.39 days compared with 5.17 days; $P = .007$). The 1-minute Apgar scores were $P < 0.0003$ and the 5-minute Apgar scores were $P < 0.00005$.

These findings are similar to the study by August (1960) where hypnoanesthesia was successful as the sole anesthetic in 93.5% of all deliveries and in eight of the 14 (57%) on caesarian sections.

In a randomized, controlled study of labor and delivery among prenatal patients, Martin et al. (2001) studied the effects of hypnosis on the labor processes and birth outcomes of pregnant adolescents using a hypnotic child-birth protocol.

Results were obtained for 22 patients in the hypnosis group and 20 in the control group, resulting in a total of 42 subjects. Only one patient in the hypnosis group had a hospital stay of more that two days compared with eight patients in the control group (P = .008). None of the 22 patients in the hypnosis group experienced surgical intervention compared with 12 of the 20 patients in the control group (P = .001). Twelve patients in the hypnosis group experienced complications compared with 17 in the control group (P = .047). Although consistently fewer patients in the hypnosis group used anesthesia (10 vs. 14), Pitocin (2 vs. 6), or postpartum medication (7 vs. 11), and fewer infants were admitted to the NICU (1 vs. 5), statistical analysis was not significant.

The hypnosis suggestions were designed to increase the patient's sense of trust in her physician and her confidence in her own ability to manage anxiety and discomfort. Ego-strengthening and suggestions paved the way for a relatively discomfort-free delivery. Although there have been numerous reports suggesting the value of hypnosis in obstetrics, our study is one of the first to report a randomized controlled evaluation of childbirth preparation incorporating hypnotic techniques on labor processes and birth outcomes (Martin et al., 2001).

A systematic meta-analyses review of hypnosis for pain relief in labor and childbirth by Cyna et al. (2004) showed the following results: Five RCTs and 14 non-randomized comparisons (NRCs) studying 8,395 women were identified where hypnosis was used for labor analgesia. Four RCTs including 224 patients examined the primary outcomes of interest. One RCT rated poor quality assessment. Meta-analyses of the (n = 189) three remaining RCTs showed that, compared with controls, fewer parturients having hypnosis required analgesia, relative risk = 0.51 (95% confidence interval 0.28, 0.95). Of the two included NRCs, one showed that women using hypnosis rated their labor pain less severe than controls (P < 0.01). The other showed that hypnosis reduced opioid (meperidine) requirements (P < 0.001), and increased the incidence of not requiring pharmacological analgesia in labor (P < 0.001) (Cyna et al., 2004).

Their primary outcome measures were labor analgesia requirements (no analgesia, opiate, or epidural use), and pain scores in labor. Suitable comparative studies were included for further assessment according to predefined criteria. Meta-analyses were performed of the included randomized controlled trials (RCTs), assessed as being of "good" or "adequate" quality by a predefined score.

Hypnosis has been utilized effectively where epidural analgesia is contraindicated, and is claimed to block all subjective perceptions of pain during labor in up to 25% of parturients. The responsiveness of women to hypnosis appears to be increased in pregnancy. In view of widespread claims of efficacy, we aimed to review the available evidence regarding the effects of hypnosis, when used for pain relief, during labor and childbirth. Women receiving hypnosis reported greater satisfaction when used for pain management in labor compared with control (RR 2.33, 95% CI 1.55 to 4.71). No differences were seen for women receiving aromatherapy, music, or audio analgesia (Cyna et al., 2004).

This report represents the most comprehensive review of the literature to date on the use of hypnosis for analgesia during childbirth. The meta-analysis shows that hypnosis reduces analgesia requirements in labor. Apart from the analgesia and anesthetic effects possible in receptive subjects, there are three other possible reasons why analgesic consumption during childbirth might be reduced when using hypnosis. First, teaching self-hypnosis facilitates patient autonomy and a sense of control. Second, the majority of parturients are likely to be able to use hypnosis for relaxation, thus reducing apprehension that in turn may reduce analgesic requirements. Finally, the possible reduction in the need for pharmacological augmentation of labor when hypnosis is used for childbirth may minimize the incidence of uterine hyperstimulation and the need for epidural analgesia.

This is a reprint from a Cochrane review on complementary and alternative therapies for pain management in labor, prepared and maintained by the Cochrane Collaboration and published in The Cochrane Library (Smith et al., 2003). Seven trials involving 366 women and using different modalities of pain management were included in this review; three studies comparing the use of hypnosis with a control group were included in the review (Freeman et al., 1986; Harmon et al., 1990; Martin et al., 2001). One trial reported on maternal satisfaction for pain relief.

All three trials reported on use of pharmacological pain relief in labor. In the Freeman trial, there was no difference in the use of pain relief between women receiving hypnosis and the control group (RR 0.88, 95% CI 0.33 to 2.24 [65 women]). In the Martin (2001) trial women receiving hypnosis used less anesthesia than women in the control group (RR 0.65, 95% CI 0.38 to 111) [42 women]). Harmon (1990) reported on the use of narcotics: fewer women in the hypnosis group used narcotics than in the control group (RR 0.21, 95% CI 0.08 to 0.55 [60 women]).

Two trials reported on spontaneous vaginal delivery (Freeman et al., 1986; Harmon et al., 1990). They found more women had a spontaneous vaginal delivery in the hypnosis group than in the control group (RR 1.38, 95% CI 1.13 to 2.47 [125 women]). Freeman (1986) found no difference in instrumental delivery between groups (RR 0.56, 95% CI 0.22 to 1.44 [65 women]).

Current evidence suggests hypnosis may be effective in reducing pain in labor. Maternal satisfaction with pain management was greater among women receiving hypnosis. Although the three included trials reported reduced use of a pharmacological pain relief in labor, when adjustive for heterogeneity between trials there was insufficient evidence of reduced use of pain relief among women receiving hypnosis. Other promising benefits from hypnosis appear to be increased vaginal delivery, and reduced use of oxytocin. One trial reported an increased duration of labor among women receiving hypnosis. There was no evidence of any adverse effects on the neonate. Further research is required (Smith et al., 2003).

Jenkins and Pritchard (1993) did a study to assess the effects of hypnosis on the first and second stages of labor in a large group of pregnant women. Included were 126 primigravid women with 200 matched controls and 136 parous women having their second baby with 300 matched controls. Only women with spontaneous deliveries were included. The hypnosis was carried on by Jenkins, who was not present at the labor.

Significantly more hypnotized primigravid women required no analgesia compared with controls (33/126 versus 13/300, respectively; $X^2 = 42$, P < 0.001). Also, significantly more hypnotized primigravid women did not require pethidine compared with controls (66/126 versus 49/300, respectively; $X^2 = 42$, P < 0.001).

Significantly more hypnotized parous women required no analgesia compared with controls (50/136 vs. 33/300, respectively; $X^2 = 32$, P < 0.001). Also, significantly more hypnotized parous women did not require pethidine compared with controls (80/136 vs. 99/300, respectively; $X^2 = 15$, P < 0.001). The use of analgesic agents was significantly reduced (P < 0.001) in both hypnotized groups compared with their controls. Harmon et al. (1990) measured obstetric outcomes and reported data on the use of medication, length of labor (stages 1 and 2), and type of delivery. Apgar scores at 1-minute and 5-minute postpartum were also recorded by one of the five referring obstetricians who delivered the baby (Apgar, 1953). The Apgar is a composite rating of the neonate's physical condition on the basis of five criteria: heart rate, respiration, muscle tone, reflex irritability, and skin color. Each criterion is rated on a scale of 0–2 with an optimum composite score of 10.

They compared labor pain with the mean pain threshold scores for hypnosis and control subjects for the ischemic pain task (Smith et al., 1966). Hypnotically trained subjects had higher pain thresholds than control subjects during sessions 3 and 4, $F (1, 58) = 18.08$, $p < .001$, and 5 and 6, $F(1, 58) = 58.60$, $p < .001$. Regardless of treatment condition, highly susceptible women had higher pain thresholds than less susceptible women during sessions 3 and 4, $F (1, 58)$

= 30.38, $p < .001$; and sessions 5 and 6, $F(1, 58) = 56.40$, $p < .001$. There was no significant three-way interaction in this analysis.

## Obstetric Outcomes

Four dependent variables were included in the ANOVA for obstetric outcomes: lengths of stage 1 and stage 2 labor and Apgar scores at 1 minute and 5 minute. There was a significant multivariate main effect of treatment condition on obstetric outcomes, $F (4, 53) = 8.29$, $p < .001$. The other multivariate main effect of susceptibility and the multivariate interaction were nonsignificant. Subsequent ANOVA tests indicated that hypnotic training was associated with shorter stage 1 labors, $F (1, 56) = 35.24$, $p < .001$, and higher Apgar scores at 1 and 5 minutes, $Fs (1, 56) = 31.37$ and $16.43$, respectively, $ps < .001$. Hypnotically prepared women had more spontaneous deliveries than control women, $X^2 (1, N = 60) = 4.69$, $p < .05$. Also, fewer hypnotically trained women received medication, $X^2 (1, N = 60) = 16.07$, $p < .001$. Specifically, compared with hypnotically trained women, larger proportions of control women received tranquilizers, $X^2 (1, N = 60) = 11.47$, $p < .001$; narcotics, $X^2 (1, N = 60) = 13.78$, $p < .001$; and oxytocics (used to stimulate contractions), $X^2 (1, N = 60) + 25.91$, $p < .001$.

In summary, we found that hypnosis resulted in shorter stage 1 labors, less medication, more spontaneous deliveries, and higher Apgar scores.

In a randomized trial of self-hypnosis for analysis in labor, Freeman et al. (1986) evaluated 29 patients in the hypnosis group and 36 in the control group. Overall, 17 of the 65 women received epidural analgesia. The incidence of normal deliveries was lower in women who received epidurals (3/17 (18%)) than in those who did not (39/48 (82%); $X^2 = 6.25$, $p < 0.01$). There was no difference in the proportion of women given epidural analgesia between the hypnosis and control groups. Good or moderate subjects had fewer epidurals (4/24) than did poor subjects (4/5; $p < 0.01$) (Freeman, 1986).

In a nonrandomized trial of self-hypnosis Davidson (1962) assessed hypnosis effect on 70 pregnant women. This was done with two main purposes: (1) to allow the patient to enjoy her pregnancy and labor; (2) to assess the effect, if any, of mental and physical relaxation on the course of labor and the need for chemical analgesia. The 70 women were taught autohypnosis in pregnancy, and the subjective sensations and objective findings in this group were compared with 70 patients taught physiotherapy relaxation through exercises and controlled breathing, and 70 control patients with no special antenatal training. In all three groups, 45 were primigravidae and 25 multigravidae. The antenatal training consisted of six "lessons" in the autohypnosis and physiotherapy relaxation sessions. The control group had the usual prenatal care.

The results showed the hypnosis group, although an older age-group by five years, and selected because of fear and anxiety, had a labor of just over half the average length of the other two groups, the average baby's weight being almost the same in each group. Although this is not a large group the reduction in the duration of labor is statistically significant ($P < 0.05$). Perhaps the greatest subjective gain was that in the autohypnosis group: 70% described the labor as pleasant, whereas only 23% of the physiotherapy patients and 33% of the controls looked back on labor as pleasant.

In conclusion, a statistically significant reduction in the duration of the first stage of labor occurred in the autohypnosis-trained group as compared with the other two groups ($P < 0.001$). Autohypnosis was found to be an effective analgesic in labor: 59% of this group of patients required no chemical analgesia in any stage of labor, whereas in the control group only 1.4% required no analgesic drug, and in the physiotherapy group all patients required some chemical analgesia. Statistically, this difference was very significant ($P < 0.001$) (Davidson, 1962).

An investigation by Mairs (1995) was done to measure differences in experiences of childbirth specifically in relation to pain, between women who had been trained in self-hypnosis and those who had not. Results showed subjects using hypnosis reported experiencing less pain during the birth of their baby. The mean pain rating for the hypnosis group during delivery was 5.86 (n = 28, S.D. 3.04) and that for the control group was 7.3 (n = 27, S.D. 2.64; Mann Whitney U, $z = -2.01$, $P = 0.045$). When the caesarean section subjects were removed (six in the hypnosis group and one in the control group), the mean pain rating for the hypnosis group during delivery was 5.41 (n = 22, S.D. 2.7) and that for the control group was 7.58 (n = 26, S.D. 2.25; Mann Whitney U, $z = -2.98$, $P = 0.003$); that is, the level of statistical significance in pain rating between groups increased.

Taking the two main groups as a whole, subjects using hypnosis reported less anxiety during the birth of their babies (post-birth reports). The mean anxiety score during birth for the hypnosis group was 5.43 (n = 28, S.D. 2.33) and for the control group 7.63 (n = 27, S.D. 1.67; Mann Whitney U, $z = -3.45$, $P = 0.0006$). With caesarean section deliveries removed, the hypnosis group mean anxiety rating during birth was 5.18 (n = 22, S.D. 2.22) and the control group 7.62 (n = 26, S.D., 1.7), which represents an increased difference between the two groups (Mann Whitney U, $z = -3.62$, $P = 0.0003$). The hypnosis group that had caesarian section deliveries (n = 6) did not differ significantly in their anxiety ratings during birth compared with either the control group (n = 27) or the hypnosis group having normal deliveries (n = 22) (Mairs, 1995). The results from this study clearly show that the use of self-hypnosis in childbirth can significantly reduce the perception of pain.

# Evidence-Based Hypnosis Use in Prevention and Treatment of Preterm Labor

Hypnosis can play a very important role in prevention of prematurity. Premature delivery of infants is the major cause of fetal loss in North America. Newton et al. (1979) showed that those pregnancies resulting in premature labor were far more common in pregnancies complicated by higher levels of psychosocial stress. Omer (1987) and others have shown that hypnosis combined with conventional pharmacologic therapy can significantly prolong the duration of pregnancies threatened by premature labor. Omer found that adding hypnosis to the treatment regimen prolonged pregnancies by an average of 18.8% longer than patients treated with medication alone.

# Empirical and Theoretical Rationale for the use of Hypnosis in Preterm Labor

Collins and Bleyl (1990), in a study of 71 quadruplet pregnancies, reported that fetal growth progressed in a linear fashion until 32 weeks' gestation. Then it slowed. The number of "growth-retarded" fetuses (< 10th percentile) dramatically increased at 34 weeks: Less than one-fourth of the fetuses are below the 10th percentile before 34 weeks, whereas 62% are below that level thereafter.

Brown and Massarelli (2002) present a case report of hypnosis use in quadruplets. The article has two purposes: First, it illustrates how medical hypnosis can be used in multiple pregnancies to assist the mother in several ways. It may help to prolong the pregnancy and to overcome the mother's feelings of incompetence about nurturing the fetuses effectively. It also deals with personal discomfort. The article's second purpose is to provide transcripts (presented in block quotations) of selected hypnosis techniques used in the reported case. The hypnotic interventions dealt with a number of the unique problems of multiple pregnancies, such as the distressing stretching pain and discomfort of the skin over the large abdomen. Hypnosis was used to minimize distress and increase the probability of prolonging the pregnancy to 32 weeks (Brown & Masserelli, 2002).

In the first trance at 24 weeks' gestation following total body relaxation, we focused on the uterus as a big muscle of longitudinal fibers, on letting them grow fast and relaxed with all the influence of hormones improving the stretching of each longitudinal fiber in order to provide more room for the four fetuses to grow normally. The profound relaxation response was used to relax the uterine vessels to improve circulation through the placenta so the fetuses would get more nourishment (facilitated by a high-calorie diet and frequent meals). The trance was facilitated at 27 weeks' gestation.

*Healing Objectives*
Improve sore buttocks from betamethazone injections; Pain relief through glove anesthesia that was then was transferred to the injection sites. The trance was carried out at 29 weeks' gestation.


*Healing Objectives*
Improve GI symptoms and improve tight skin across the front of the abdomen by stretching skin from back around both sides.


**Script for Abdominal Enlargement**
"A whirlpool bath will help your body create space for the uterus to enlarge… Imagine the uterine wall like a piece of clay that as you warm it up to just the right temperature, can stretch a little bit easier so you can feel your skin warming and stretching normally, slowly, without any tearing – just stretching and responding to the pregnancy as you get into the thirties [30 weeks' of gestation]. You will find… that soothing warm whirlpool bath will also soothe the uterine muscle, so it will be relaxed and any irritation will be flushed away with the whirlpool so the muscle will be placid…"

Hypnosis is an excellent way to reduce and even prevent stress prenatally as well as during labor and delivery. Numerous authors have noted that under hypnosis, women are relaxed, show less postpartum exhaustion, and feel surprisingly well after the delivery (Brown & Murphy, 1999). Lederman (1995) discusses cognitive and behavioral strategies including hypnotic relaxation for decreasing anxiety and promoting relaxation during gestation and parturition. These studies show that stress plays an important role in increasing the risk of preterm labor (Brown & Murphy, 1999). There have been no randomized controlled clinical trials comparing the relative effectiveness of medical hypnosis therapy with the usual therapy for preterm labor.

Another remarkable result of the trances occurred after the fifth session. At 29 weeks' gestation, with a fundal height of 49 cm, her abdominal skin was too tight to possibly stretch any further. Suggestions were made, using the metaphor of a warm whirlpool bath that the skin, tissues, and muscles of the abdominal wall would stretch in all directions, including around from the back. After that, her girth dramatically increased over a short period of time, so that several nurses who had been caring for her during her hospital stay commented on the change.

There were three other particularly helpful aspects of the trances:

1. The use of anatomically precise terms was important because of the patient's knowledge as a physician. "…practice relaxing and stretching those muscle fibers and stretching all the tissues of the uterus…the endocervical area and the cervical canal as it gets longer too…and the inner ring of the cervix can relax some, but the outer ring, the exocervix as you noted, it has been reported to you as staying competent and it will continue to stay competent…it will remain tightly closed as your longitudinal uterine muscles and fibers stretch and the uterus gets larger…you can be really proud of yourself…"

2. The observation, during the trances, of normal events like increased fetal movement (which was routinely experienced) as sources of positive feedback, and its use for ego-strengthening, was very helpful.

3. Phrasing the unique circumstances of this pregnancy positively, as in "one day is equal to four baby-days, so you are doing well…" and "…you will think of the four neonatal teams just as a normal procedure for someone having four babies at once…so they are all part of the team…" was a good way to allay anxiety.

Because multiple gestations result in a large number of preterm deliveries, there is a great need for clinical trials on the use of hypnosis in multiple gestations. The best way to answer the question, "Does hypnosis make a difference?" is by doing a large multicenter randomized controlled clinical trial. Much more research is needed to answer this question for both singleton and multiple gestations.

Hypnosis treats preterm labor on several levels. First, patients learn to control the psychosocial stress of pregnancy. Second, hypnosis can be used to teach the patient to be more aware of contractions, and therefore initiate pharmacologic therapy at an earlier, more effective point in the pregnancy. Third, the relaxation effect of hypnosis not only makes tolerance of the pharmacologic agents easier (agents such as ritodrine and terbutaline have stimulant effects), but also serves to relax the uterine muscle, directly reducing the probability of premature labor. Hypnosis can also increase the patient's motivation to continue the pregnancy to term through imagery focusing on the delivery of a full term healthy infant. The extra attention and social support given to patients taught by hypnosis may also contribute to the reduction in prematurity rates noted (Goldman, 1992).

Schwartz (1963) reported the cessation of labor in three patients using hypnotic techniques. In the first patient he was able to have her stop preterm labor a number of times to prolong the pregnancy from 29 weeks' gestation to 32 weeks to deliver a more mature live infant. In the second case, Mrs LH was able to stop her labor in spite of the fact that she was almost completely dilated until her doctor delivered another patient. He returned 30 minutes later and suggested she start contracting again. She promptly resumed labor and within ten minutes the head was crowning. In the third case, the woman at term in labor developed acetone in her urine and was tired. She was given IV glucose and told to stop her contractions; she then stopped contractions again to be moved for delivery, and a nine-pound breech infant was born. A complete perineoplasty was done using only hypnoanesthesia. The use of hypnosis in the stopping of labor in both premature and full-term labors has been illustrated by these cases.

Logan (1963) also reported three cases where hypnosis was used to delay labor. Case one presented on July 22 and admitted to hospital at seven months' gestation with abdominal cramps and recurrent vaginal bleeding. Early in this pregnancy, her second child died of aspirin poisoning at the age of 22 months. On July 24 the author was asked to see the patient in consultation. Hypnosis was induced on three successive days and the patient was discharged on July 27. She was readmitted on October 6 at term, in labor, and delivered a healthy male infant.

The second woman presented at the hospital at 27 weeks' gestation in active labor. After 24 hours, consultation hypnosis was started. Suggestions were given that, since she was not at term, she would stop having contractions and wait until the proper time, that is, until her expected date of confinement. Within 15 minutes, the uterine contractions slowed down and then ceased. She was discharged from the hospital the next day. She returned to the hospital at term in March 1962.

In the third case, a 23-year-old Gr IV para III had a due date of June 28. This date coincided with an International Congress on Obstetrics and Gynecology, which this patient's obstetrician wished to attend. On May 9 under hypnosis the following suggestions were given: "When you have your baby in two months time" followed by the other usual suggestions for preparation for labor and delivery. The patient went into labor while the author was attending the meeting. She reported later that "something kept telling" her that this was "not the time to be in labor," so after three hours her contractions stopped. On July 8 she was seen at a regular prenatal visit. On examination she was four centimeters dilated with bulging membranes, but she was not having any contractions. An after-hours appointment was arranged at the hospital for the patient where she was hypnotized and given permission to go into labor. One hour later she delivered a healthy female infant.

The first study in the literature that reported comparing hypnosis use in premature labor cases with controls that received medications alone was done by Hiam Omer (1987).

His paper describes hypnotic relaxation techniques that proved effective in prolonging pregnancy in a sample of 39 patients hospitalized for premature labor. Seventy-four women hospitalized with the same diagnosis in the same ward served as a control group. All of the women were between their 26th and 34th week of pregnancy. Women in both groups received the standard pharmacological treatment for premature labor. The comparison was between a group receiving medications alone and a group receiving hypnotherapy in addition to medication.

Hypnotic-relaxation was administered by the author. In 38 cases treatment was started within 3 hours of hospitalization, and in the remaining case within 14 hours of hospitalization. Treatment lasted for 3 hours on the average: 90 minutes in the first meeting and another 90 minutes during the following days. Apart from the treatment administered in person, each woman had an audiocassette of a hypnotic exercise especially recorded for her. She was told to exercise with the cassette twice daily during her hospital stay and once daily at home until the end of her 37th pregnancy week. His paper presents a detailed description of the hypnotic intervention.

The patient was told that the goal of this hypnotic-relaxation exercise was to relax her whole body and her uterus in particular. Ideomotor finger questioning was done to see if there was a readiness in the subconscious mind to carry the pregnancy to 37 weeks. There were 34 positive answers, two negatives and three no answers. The main dependent variable was the Rate of Pregnancy Prolongation (RPP), which was defined as follows: RRP = (lag time between onset of treatment and day of delivery/lag time between onset of treatment and expected day of delivery) × 100%. The average infant weight in the two groups was also compared.

Results showed a significant superiority for the hypnotic group. Mean RPP for this group was 75.2%, whereas mean RPP for the control group was 55.4% (Student's $t = 3.09$, $p < 0.002$, $df = 111$). Mean infant weight for the hypnotic group was 2917 g and for the control group, 2692 g (Student's $t = 1.64$, $p = 0.05$, $df = 111$).

Short-term hypnotherapy contrasts deeply with many medical innovations, which may achieve treatment effects only at a very high cost in terms of technology, hospitalization, expensive diagnostic procedures, etc.

Hypnotherapy was shown to be effective as an adjunct to the medical treatment of premature labor.

David Cheek (1995) has given the most lucid picture of early use of psychotherapy in prevention of preterm labor. Conscious and unconscious fears appear to be the cause of preterm labor. The hypothesis is presented that pyramiding maternal fear starts a sequence of events that can culminate in expulsive preterm labor when premature infants conclude that they are not wanted. An important feature of treatment is the re-establishment of maternal–fetal telepathic communications that are stopped when a pregnant woman loses hope of having a living child.

The incidence of preterm deliveries in my practice between 1946 and 1956 was 6.8% in spite of my knowledge that emotional factors were involved in each case. Verbal reassurance and hypnotic relaxation made no difference. My fetal mortality from prematurity was about the same as that of my colleagues in a similar practice at that time. The factors responsible for preterm labor lay below conscious awareness and were not reached by verbal interchange. After incorporating use of ideomotor search methods with hypnosis in my final 12 years of clinical obstetrical practice, my incidence of preterm births dropped to 2.6% and all my premature babies weighed more than four pounds; all survived.

There is an underlying pattern of development in the sequence of events leading to a change from painless Braxton Hicks contractions to those starting at the two horns of the uterus and progressing downward to dilate the cervix and expel the fetus. This became clear during my research on the unconscious factors in preterm labor:

1.  The pregnant woman becomes unconsciously alarmed about the safety of her infant.

2.  She has recurring troubled dreams that are not remembered on awakening.

3.  She is awakened eventually by painful contractions that previously have occurred unnoticed. These are initially only painful concentric contractions. They continue to squeeze out used blood and allow ingress of fresh blood carrying oxygen to the fetus and will not threaten the fetus unless the mother panics.

4.  But a pregnant woman will be alarmed because recurring pains mean labor to her at a time that would endanger her unborn infant. She will report her distress to her midwife or obstetrician.

5.  Her midwife or obstetrician will be afraid that inaction might be interpreted as malpractice in the event that a premature infant is born.

Active treatment increases the patient's apprehension and thus contributes to a continuation of painful Braxton Hicks contractions. Realization that none of the treatments are relieving her pain makes the pregnant women stop communicating with her fetus. Fetal–maternal telepathic communication is an innate bonding process used by all happily pregnant women. It stops if the woman feels she may not be able to have that baby.

The premature fetus will secrete messenger proteins that transfer the placenta into the maternal circulation to trigger the mother's release of prostaglandins and oxytocin. Labor begins (McDonald & Nathanielsz, 1991; Nathanielsz, 1992, 1994).

The process from initial distress to the time of beginning expulsive labor may take a few hours for a particularly distressed pregnant woman but usually is measured in days or weeks before the fetus or fetuses become troubled enough to start their mother into labor. The sequence can be stopped at any time with combined hypnoanalytic techniques between the beginning and the moment fetal membranes have ruptured or the cervix has dilated beyond four centimeters.

One or both fetuses eventually become alarmed because the mother is not normally active. She is on bed rest with the constant companion of a uterine monitor. It senses her anxiety and her telepathic silence as indicative of not wanting to be pregnant.

## Psychological Intervention

Women whose unconscious fears have been addressed and removed during the first trimester are not likely to go into premature labor.

Most obstetricians, however, do not use hypnosis to explore prenatal and birth imprintings that can strongly influence a woman's attitude toward childbearing.

Intervention usually starts after the above train of events has begun. The work is easy if the first telephone call occurs before the frightened patient has contacted her midwife or doctor. It becomes progressively more difficult after active treatment has begun. Intervention after effacement and beginning dilation of the cervix requires a constant vigil and repeated calls to ensure safe conduct for the remainder of the pregnancy. The concern and interactions of innocent friends and relatives can overturn otherwise constructive therapy.

The two cases reported here are excellent examples of relatively easy intervention. Three telephone calls were all that were needed for the first case and seven with the second, more vulnerable patient. Both women had read about emotional factors initiating preterm labor.

David Cheek (1995) presents two excellent examples of women in preterm labor verbatim in such a way that the reading clinician gains insight and learns what to say and how to manage preterm labor patients successfully with comfort for both the patient and the physician. Helpful information is also found in Brown & Murphy (1999) and Brown & Massarelli (2002) and Omer (1987).

## Comment

Again a problem was created by apprehensive doctors and friends. Continuing worry could have eventuated in true preterm labor. Betty's understanding about the mechanisms of Braxton Hicks contractions helped raise her tolerance for pain. Of great help in this instance was her innate and constant communications with her twins. Her realization that dreams can be responsible for complications was helpful, as was the recognition of her husband's full emotional support.

Lou et al. (1992) reports on psychosocial stress and severe prematurity. In prematurity, a significant correlation was obtained only for psychological stressful events (p = 0.015, DSM III R axis four, grades 4 and 5). The attributable fraction was 11%. Fatigue at work did not contribute measurably. Suboptimum schooling (under 11 years), smoking, and daily alcohol intake contributed with 14, 13, and 1.5%, respectively, to the Intra Uterine Growth Retardation (IUGR) group (p = 0.047, p = 0.0095, and p = 0.038). Thus, psychosocial stress was a risk factor for severe prematurity.

Hedegaard et al. (1993) investigated psychological distress during pregnancy and its relation risk of preterm delivery. Their *Design* was a prospective, population based, follow-up study with repeated measures of psychological distress, based on the use of questionnaires. Data from the 30th week showed a strong association between distress and preterm delivery. The risk of preterm delivery rose gradually from about 1% for low scores to about 6% for high scores in a dose-response relation.

The conclusions included that psychological distress later in pregnancy is associated with an increased risk of preterm delivery. Future interventional studies should focus on ways of lowering psychological distress in late pregnancy.

Newton (1989) reported the influence of psychosocial stress in low birth weight and preterm labor in a prospective study where he confirmed that there was a significant association between the experience of major life events and preterm delivery (p < 0.001). Mutale et al. (1991) did a study of life events, stress, and low birth weight. Social stress was assessed in 92 women with low-birth weight babies and 92 controls using the detailed LEDS measure of life events and severe chronic difficulties. The low-birth weight group was divided into preterm delivery (n = 40), small for gestational age (SGA) (n = 40), and mixed groups. Comparison of preterm births with controls indicated that three factors were significantly associated: a previous low-birth weight baby, severe life event/difficulty, and bleeding during pregnancy. By using a reliable measure of life events and adequate numbers of low-birth weight babies, this study overcame the potential inaccuracies of previous studies and indicates a more specific relation between social stress and low birth weight.

The variables that emerged as significant were: previous low-birth weight baby (p < 0.001), severe life event and/or difficulty (p < 0.001), and bleeding during pregnancy (p < 0.001). Even after these three factors had been accounted for there was a further significant effect attributable to severe life events/chronic difficulties during pregnancy for the preterm group. Whereas Newton & Hunt (1984) found an effect of events and difficulties during the last trimester, the present study found the effect was related to severe life events and difficulties throughout pregnancy. This was a surprising finding since an increase in catecholamine excretion, associated with social stress during the last trimester, has been postulated as a trigger of preterm labor.

Papiernik et al. (1986) began a longitudinal study in France in 1971 and continued for 12 years, a total of 16,004 singleton pregnancies were followed. Preterm deliveries (<37 weeks) fell from 6.3% in 1971–74, to 4.6% in 1975–78 and 4.2% 1979–82. P < 0.001. Low-birth weight deliveries (<2,500 g) dropped from 5.2% in 1971–74, to 4.3% in 1975–78 and 4.2% in 1979–82. P < 0.05.

The recognition that heavy work is causally related to preterm delivery was confirmed by a prospective study of 3,500 women from the cities of Haguenau and Lyon by Mamelle et al. (1981).

Luke et al. (1995) reported a study on the association between occupational factors and preterm birth in nurses in the United States. Factors significantly associated with preterm birth included hours worked per week (p < 0.002), per shift (p < 0.001), and while standing (p < 0.001); noise (p = 0.005); physical exertion (p = 0.01); and occupational fatigue score (p < 0.002). The adjusted odds ratios were 1.6 (p = 0.006) for hours worked per week (36 vs. >36) and 1.4 (p = 0.02) for fatigue score < 3 vs. 3.

Among the conclusions were that preterm birth among working women may be related to hours worked per day or week and to adverse working conditions.

Copper et al. (1996) report on their preterm prediction study: Maternal stress is associated with spontaneous preterm birth at less than 35 weeks' gestation. Their purpose was to determine whether various measures of poor psychosocial status in pregnancy are associated with spontaneous preterm birth, fetal growth restriction, or low birth weight.

Anxiety, stress, self-esteem, mastery, and depression were assessed at 25 to 29 weeks in 2,593 gravid women by use of a 28-item Likert scale. Their scale was an adaptation of five previously validated tools that measure trait anxiety, self-esteem, mastery, depression, and stress. In their analysis a score indicating high stress was significantly associated with spontaneous preterm birth (5.3% vs. 3.0%, p = 0.003) and LBW (13.5% vs. 9.6%, p = 0.003). No other psychosocial characteristic was significantly associated with spontaneous preterm birth, IUGR, or LBW. For the most part, obstetric interventions aimed at the prevention of LBW or its components, spontaneous preterm birth or IUGR, have been unsuccessful. They stated that further study is needed to determine whether psychosocial and behavioral interventions during pregnancy are beneficial.

Lederman (1995) reviewed articles with a focus on recent research that examined the relationship among the major types of stressors, anxiety, and development of maternal, fetal, and neonatal problems or complications.

The research literature covering both human and animal species shows that maternal stress, by activating abnormally high levels of peptides (e.g., adrenocorticotrophic hormone (ACTH) and beta-endorphin β-E) from the hypothalamic-pituitary-adrenal (HPA) axis, influences fetal growth, central nervous system development and behavior, and neonatal birth outcomes in profound and long-lasting ways. The increase in β-E levels were also associated with decreased uteroplacental blood flow resulting in fetal hypoxia, which was attributed to maternal stress.

From the foregoing, it can be seen that multidimensional measures of stress are warranted in the analysis of reproductive health outcomes. They have been advocated elsewhere as well. Two other reviews of the literature of stress and birth outcomes have concluded that life-event stress is most consistently correlated with prenatal events, particularly with preterm delivery or gestational age (prematurity), rather than with complications during delivery. Others have shown that cortisol reactivity and anxiety are also related to premature birth.

Mamelle et al. (1989) describe both the development of and results of the use of a self-administered questionnaire designed specifically to investigate the relation between the psychological attitudes of pregnant women toward pregnancy and an eventual subsequent premature birth. The questionnaire was used in a prospective survey. A quantitative PPAT(p) score (ranging from 0 to 6) was constructed in a working sample (n = 643), and its relation with a subsequent premature birth was analyzed in a study sample (n = 1,500). The risk of premature birth increased from 1 to 1.5 when the PPAT(p) score increased one point (p < 0.001). This study contributes to a better understanding of psychologic factors that may affect pregnant women and be associated with premature birth. The questionnaire was easily completed in about 20 minutes by a large number subjects.

Williamson et al. (1989) measured the association between stressful life changes, social supports, and serious complications of pregnancy in 513 women obtaining prenatal care in four rural family practices. Those women whose life-change score (LCS) increased from the second to the third trimester had a significantly higher rate of poor outcomes (neonatal death, transfer to a neonatal intensive care unit, birthweight less than 2,500 g or 5-minute Apgar score less than 7) than those whose LCS did not increase (9.2% vs. 3.9%, P = 0.015). This effect of increasing stress was present even after controlling for demographic and standard obstetric risk factors. High life change scores at 20 weeks' gestation and 34 weeks' gestation were not individually associated with poor outcomes. A one-time finding of high stress was not a predictor of poor outcome, but a progressive increase in stressful life change was associated with adverse outcome. Some aspects of this study are unique. First, the effect of stress was shown to be independent of biomedical risk by logistic regression. Second, this study used only clinically important perinatal morbidity as criteria in defining poor outcome.

Most important, this study showed that serious, clinically significant complications of pregnancy can be related to stressful life changes independent of biomedical risk.

Brown and Murphy (1999) report two pilot projects using hypnosis to treat preterm labor. The first pilot project objectives were to develop the methodologies, a hypnosis script, and a PGFM radioimmunoassay.

Hypnosis started within six hours after informed consent was received. She was given suggestions in trance to keep her cervix firm and hard to hold her baby in the uterus. Hypnosis was continued until labor stopped. Later at the patient's convenience, she was given a specific hypnosis stress treatment program to fit her internal map. Audiotapes were made of her trances and she was requested to listen to them at least twice daily while in hospital.

Negative birth experiences (Barnett, 1989) were modified to positive ones and each patient was assessed for any unconscious fears for this and other pregnancies utilizing ideomotor questioning methods (Rossi & Cheek, 1998). Thus, any unconscious fears were resolved by reframing. As long as the contractions continued, the hypnotherapist visited the patient two or three times per day. The hypnotherapist checked on the patient daily while she remained in hospital.

After discharge, the patient was advised to listen to the tape at least once daily until she reached 37 weeks' gestation. She kept a daily record of trances and the number of times she listened to audiotapes on a time date record.

## Evaluation of the Effectiveness of Hypnosis

The effectiveness of the hypnosis was measured using the following parameters:

1.   The primary outcome measure was gestation at delivery.

2.   Cessation of premature labor and prolongation of pregnancy.

3.   Health status of the neonate, based on birth weight, Apgar score, and the length of time spent in the neonatal intensive care unit, time on respirator.

4.   The length of hospital stay for mother and babies.

The second measure was that described by Omer (1987) and colleagues, who developed a rate of pregnancy prolongation (RPP) scale in 1985, and demonstrated that it could fulfil the criteria of high sensitivity to treatment and of unbiasedness for the gestational patients.

All women admitted to the Grace Maternity Hospital, Halifax, NS, with the diagnosis of preterm labor were considered for the first study.

Patients that gave informed consent were able to choose the hypnosis therapy group or the usual therapy nonhypnosis group. The hypnosis group received the usual therapy for premature labor plus hypnosis.

During the first pilot project, nine patients in preterm labor agreed to have hypnosis.

Total number of patients in the study was 35: hypnosis 9, control 2, and 24 term labor patients. Clinical findings (e.g., rate of pregnancy prolongation) are reported in Table 1. Gestation at delivery and birth weight are reported in Table 2 for the hypnosis subjects and Table 3 for the control subjects.

## Table 1: Clinical Findings

| Subject | EDC | Gestation at entry | Latency | RPP | |
|---|---|---|---|---|---|
| H-1 | Oct 2/93 | 27 weeks | 2 days = | 2 days/88 = | 2.3% |
| H-2 | May 9/94 | 24 weeks | 85 days = | 85 days/102 = | 83.3% |
| H-3 | June 2/94 | 24 weeks | 44 days = | 44 days/38 = | 100% |
| H-4 | Sept 21/94 | 19 weeks | 110 days = | 110 days/113 = | 97% |
| H-5 | Aug 22/94 | 33 weeks | 46 days = | 46 days/47 = | 97.9% |
| H-6 | Nov 10/94 | 25 weeks | 72 days = | 72 days/69 = | 100% |
| H-7 | Oct 28/94 | 25 weeks | 44 days = | 44 days/81 = | 54.3% |
| H-8 | Dec 4/94 | 28 weeks | 82 days = | 82 days/87 = | 94.2% |
| H-9 | Mar 28/95 | 25 weeks | 2 days = | 2 days/104 = | 1.9% |
| **Controls** | | | | | |
| C-1 | Sept 26/93 | 27 weeks | 1 day = | 1 day/87 = | 1.1% |
| C-2 | Oct 10/93 | 35 weeks | 12 days = | 12 days/31 = | 38.7% |

H = hypnosis C = Control RPP = Rate of Pregnancy Prolongation

Gestation at delivery and birth weight are reported in Table 2 for the hypnosis subjects and Table 3 for the control subjects.

## Table 2: Clinical Results

| | | Baby Birth | |
|---|---|---|---|
| | **Gestation at Delivery** | **Sex** | **Weight** |
| H-1 | 27–3/7 weeks | M | 1315 g |
| H-2 | 38 weeks | F | 2615 g |
| H-3 | 40 weeks | M | 2907 g |
| H-4 | 29–4/7 weeks | F | 3545 g |
| H-5 | 40 weeks | F | 3334 g |
| H-6 | 40 weeks | M | 4055 g |
| H-7 | 31–4/7 weeks | F | 2180 g |
| H-8 | 39–3/7 weeks | M | 3466 g |
| H-9 | 25–2/7 by dates | M | 461 g |
| | 23–24 weeks | M | 620 g |
| | Average Weight | | 2227 g |

## Table 3: Clinical Results

| | | Baby Birth | |
|---|---|---|---|
| **Controls** | **Gestation at Delivery** | **Sex** | **Weight** |
| C-1 | 27 weeks | F | 1095 g |
| C-2 | 36 weeks | F | 2065 g |
| | Average Weight | | 1580 g |

In summary, the mean RPP for the hypnosis patients = 70.1% (N = 9), for controls 19.9% (N = 2)

The nine hypnosis subjects included one woman with twins; a stillborn weighing 461 g and a live twin weighing 620 g. The average weight for the ten infants was 2,227 g. The average weight of two controls was 1,580 g, a difference of 647 grams. Five of the hypnosis subjects also had tocolysis. Hypnosis was successful as the sole anesthetic in 61% (22/36) of deliveries, whereas in the control group 2.7% (1/36) did not require any anesthetic or premedication.

We achieved all our objectives for the pilot projects. The hypnosis script was developed and modified. Patients had hypnosis within six hours of informed consent. More patients were recruited into the hypnosis arm than into the control arm of the study during the first pilot project. All subjects in the Australian pilot project wanted to be randomized to the hypnosis group. This speaks well for recruitment of patients into a larger randomized controlled clinical trial. There is excellent potential here for an international, multicenter, cooperative clinical trial.

Mamelle et al. (1997) did a study where the objective was to assess the effectiveness of psychological support against preterm delivery in pregnant women with symptoms of preterm labor. On the whole, the preterm delivery rate observed among the women of the experimental group was 12.3% versus 25.7% in the control group ($p < 0.01$). If the results are expressed as a relative risk of preterm birth in the experimental group compared with the control group, the estimate of crude relative risk is of 0.48 (95% confidence interval 0.34 to 0.67) across the whole sample – or the risk of preterm delivery among the women in the experimental group is one half that of the control group. This study confirms the feasibility of this kind of intervention and the effectiveness of psychological support on the risk of preterm delivery.

Picone et al. (1982) examined in a study the roles of diet, cigarette smoking, and psychological stress in pregnancy weight gain. The 60 subjects were selected by defined criteria to minimize variation in anthropometric, socioeconomic, and medical factors, which also affect weight gain. To maximize variation in weight gain, subjects were also selected on the basis of low weight gain (15lb) and adequate weight gain (>15 lb). Each weight gain group contained smokers and nonsmokers. Smokers consumed more calories than nonsmokers (2,119 vs. 1,810 kcal/day, $p < 0.01$). For nonsmokers, differences between the intakes of low weight gain (1,617 kcal/day) and adequate weight gain (1,905 kcal/day) women were significant ($p < 0.002$) and calorie intake was correlated with weight gain ($r = 0.44$, $p < 0.02$). Psychological stress negatively correlated with weight gain (= 0.37, $p < 0.01$) but not with calorie intake. Low weight gain subjects had more problems with family members ($X2 = 3.28$, $p < 0.06$), had less acceptance of their pregnancy by family members (X2 = 5.5, p < 0.02), and felt less satisfaction with their personal life (X2 = 8.6, p < 0.01).

Newton (1989) presented a modified life-events inventory over a four-month period to 132 consecutive women going into spontaneous labor. Three study groups were identified according to the duration of pregnancy. The levels of psychosocial stress in pregnancy were found to be particularly high in the mothers whose babies were born preterm. Stressful events may precipitate preterm labor in some women.

Results showed that the numbers of pregnancies in each study group were accompanied by no major life events at one end of the scale and five major life events at the other. Only 36 (43%) of the 83 mothers whose pregnancies went to term experienced any major life events compared with 20 of the 30 (67%) who went into preterm labor and 16 of the 19 (84%) whose babies were very preterm.

When the results are presented in terms of the mean number of life events per pregnancy it is apparent that the more premature the onset of labor the higher the level of psychosocial stress is likely to be. Significantly more major life events occurred in the preterm than the term group (P < 0.02), and the difference between the very preterm and the term groups was highly significant (P < 0.01).

**Tables 4 and 5 present summaries of relevant data.**

## *Table 4: Efficacious Hypnosis Use in Obstetrics Labor*

1. Bobart and Brown (2002):

    a) One-minute Apgar scores were p < 0.0003. Five-minute Apgar scores were p < 0.00005.

    b) Use of Regional Anesthesia in Labor Delivery. Regional (97%) 35 controls 35/36 had it. (38%) 14/36 hypnosis had it.

    c) Use of Analgesia in Labor Delivery. Analgesia only 5.5% of hypnosis group required it. 75% of control group required analgesia.

    d) Length of Hospital Stay. Hypnosis group 4.39 days. Controls (5.17 days) (p = 0.007)

2. August (1960) use of hypnosis. Hypnoanesthesia was successful as the sole anesthetic in 93.5 % of all deliveries and in eight of the 14 (57%) caesarian sections.

3. Martin et al. (2001) use of:

    a) Anesthesia – Hypnosis group less than control group (RR 0.65, 95% (I 0.38 to 111)) (42 women).

    b) Analgesia – Hypnosis women rated labor pain less severe than controls (p < 0.01).

    c) Surgical intervention – None of the 22 hypnosis group required vs. 12 of 20 controls (p = 0.001).

    d) Hospital stay – One hypnosis patient over two days vs. eight controls (p = 0.008).

    e) Complications – 12 of hypnosis patients and 17 in control group (p = 0.047).

4. Cyna et al. (2004) in a meta-analysis of three randomized controlled trials (RCT) s showed fewer hypnosis subjects required analgesia than controls. Relative risk + 0.51.

    a) Anesthesia – Hypnosis less than controls (RR 0.65, 95%, C1 0.38 to 111) (42 women).

    b) Hypnosis patients use less analgesia than controls. Relative risk = 0.51 (95% C1 0.28, 0.95) (p < 0.001).

    c) Use of opioid (p < 0.001).

    d) Women receiving hypnosis had greater satisfaction for pain management than controls (RR 2.33, 95%, C1 1.55 to 4.71) and they rated labor pain as less severe (p < 0.01).

5. Jenkins and Pritchard (1993):

    a) Analgesia use reduced in hypnosis patients (p < 0.001).

    b) Length of Labor – first stage primigravadas (p < 0.0001), second stage (p < 0.001). First stage parous women (p < 0.01).

    c) More hypnosis patients did not require pethidine vs. controls 66/126 vs. 49/300 (p < 0.001)

6. Freedman et al. (1986):

    a) Anesthesia – Good hypnosis subjects required fewer epidurals (p < 0.001)

    b) More women had spontaneous vaginal delivery in the hypnosis group than controls (RR 1.38 (95 C1 1.13 to 2.47 (125 women)).

7. Davidson (1962) use of:

    a) Length of labor in hypnosis group just over half the length of two control groups (p < 0.001).

    b) Analgesia – 59% of hypnosis group required *no* analgesia where as 1.4% of controls required *no* analgesia (p < 0.001).

    c) Pleasant labor – 70% of hypnosis group, only 23% of physiotherapy group and 33% of control group pleasant.

8. Mairs (1995):

    a) Level of anxiety – Hypnosis mean score 5.43 (n = 28, SD 2.33) and for the controls 7.63 (n = 27, SD 1.67) (p = 0.001). Caesarian section hypnosis group mean 5.18 (n = 22, SD 2.22) and caesarian controls group 7.62 (n = 26, SD 1.7) (p = 0.0003) (pain level).

    b) Perception of pain – Hypnosis subjects reported less pain 5.41 vs. 7.58 controls (p = 0.003).

    c) Pain rating level – Hypnosis group 5.86 (n = 28, SD3.04) control group: 7.3) (n = 27, SD 2.64) (p = 0.045).

    d) Caesarian section – Hypnosis subjects n = 6 reported less pain than control caesarian section patients (p = 0.003).

9. Harmon et al. (1990):

    a) Narcotics use – More controls used, $X^2$ (1, N = 60) = 13.87 (p < 0.001).

b) Analgesia/tranquilizer use – More controls used from $X^2$ (1, N = 60) = 11.47, p < 0.001).

c) Anesthesia – Hypnotic patients used less meds $X^2$ (1, N = 60) = 16.07 (p, 0.001).

d) Length of labor – Stage one labors F (1, 56) = 35.24 (p < 0.001).

e) Type of delivery – More hypnosis had spontaneous delivery $X^2$ (1, N = 60) 4.69 (p < 0.05).

f) Apgar scores – One minute Apgar scores hypnotic higher $F_s$ (1,56) = 31.37 and five minute 16.43 (ps < 0.001).

g) Pain threshold – Hypnosis is higher than controls F (1,58) – 18.08 (p < 0.001). Hypnosis higher than controls 5 + 6 sessions F (1, 58) = 58.60 (p < 0.001).

h) Tranquilizer use – More controls needed tranquilizers, $X^2$ (1, N = 60) = 11.47 (p < 0.001)

## Table 5: Empirical and Theoretical Rational for Hypnosis Use in Treatment and Prevention of Preterm Labor (PTL)

1) Brown and Massarelli (2002). The main objective of hypnosis was to prolong the pregnancy to 32 weeks by preventing PTL. The pregnancy was terminated at 31 weeks' gestation by caesarian section (without PTL) because of toxemia, e.g., objective was achieved and four healthy infants were delivered. All had normal weights for gestation. All are doing well as teenagers.

2) Newton (1979). PTL – level of psychosocial stress and onset of preterm labor. Only 36 (43%) of the 83 mothers delivered at term had major life events compared with 20 of 30 (67%) (p < 0.02) who had PTL and 16 of the 19 (84%) (p < 0.01) whose babies were born very preterm.

3) Omer (1987). Rate of Pregnancy Prolongation (RPP) cases vs. controls 18.8%. Results (students ± = 3.09, p < 0.002, dF 111). Hypnotic group mean infant weight 2,917 g and control infant weight 2,692 g (students = 1.64, p = 0.05, dF 111).

4) Brown and Murphy (1990). Hypnosis (N = 9) RPP = 70.1% and two controls RPP = 19.9%.

5) Luke et al. (1995). a) PT birth and (2) hours wk/wk ($p < 0.002$); b) hours per shift ($p < 0.001$); c) while standing ($p < 0.001$); d) noise ($p = 0.005$); e) physical exertion ($p = 0.01$); f) occupational fatigue ($p < 0.002$).

6) Schwartz (1963). Hypnosis in stopping preterm labor and labor at term when necessary. Reported cessation of labor in three patients with hypnosis. One stopped preterm labor a number of times to go from 29 weeks' gestation to 32 weeks' gestation to deliver a more mature infant. Two in labor at term almost completely dilated for 30 minutes until her obstetrician arrived. Third stopped because acetone (hypnosis + intravenous fluids – stopped labor) in labor and tired until in delivery room.

7) Brown and Murphy (1999). Treated nine patients in preterm labor with hypnosis and their gestation RPP was = 70.1% and for two controls 19.9%.

8) Logan (1963). Patient at seven months' gestation. Hypnosis stopped labor for three days and later delivered at term. Case 2 at 27 weeks' gestation. Hypnosis to stop labor "until the proper time." Delivered at term. Case 3 in labor at 32 weeks. Under hypnosis told "when you have baby in two months." She stopped her labor and dilated at 4 cm. Not in labor at term. Then started labor when so instructed at hospital a few hours later.

9) Cheek (1995). Risk factors in producing preterm labor.

10) Fetal messenger proteins as cause agents to trigger labor in the mother (MacDonald & Nathanielsz, 1991; Nathanielsz 1992, 1994).

11) Lou et al. (1992). Psychosocial stress and severe prematurity – showed significant $p = 0.015$.

12) Hedgeaard et al. (1993). Psychological distress later (last trimester) in pregnancy and preterm labor. Psychological distress later in pregnancy found a distinct association between distress in the 30th week gestation and risk of PT delivery. The adjusted relative risk for preterm delivery of the moderate and high categories were 1.32 (0.83 to 2.06) and 1.92 (1.23 to 3.00) comparable to the findings among all women.

13) Newton (1989). Major life events last trimester. Low birth rate $p = <0.01$, $p < 0.05$ with matched controls. Preterm delivery $p = <0.001$ PTD with matched controls $p = <0.005$.

14) Mutale (1991). a) Severe life events and low birth weight; b) Social stress throughout pregnancy; c) Previous low birth weight <0.001; d) Severe event and/or chronic difficulty <0.001; e) Bleeding during pregnancy <0.001.

# Future Developments in Research and Clinical Practice

A considerable percentage of preterm deliveries are attributed to multiple gestations. Patients in preterm labor have shown that they are eager and willing to be assigned (randomized to) to the hypnosis arm of the study.

There is a great need for a multicenter randomized controlled trial (RCT) on hypnosis use in patients in preterm labor with multiple gestations, e.g. twins, triplets, and quadruplet pregnancies, to see how big the difference in preterm delivery rate is between the hypnosis and control groups.

Among the conclusions: Significant reduction was demonstrated in labor and delivery pain and need for medication during and after labor and delivery. During the training sessions the patients are taught alternative ways to produce hypnoanalgesia and anesthesia. The hypnosis therapist is not needed at the delivery. About 60% of women using self-hypnosis can deliver without medication and anesthesia. Hypnosis was shown to be an effective adjunct to the medical treatment of preterm labor.

A multicenter randomized clinical trial of hypnosis use in singleton preterm labor patients is proposed, as is another RCT of hypnosis use to treat patients with multiple gestations (twins, triplets, and quadruplets) to prevent and evaluate preterm delivery rates. This is important because quadruplet pregnancies are now much more common and represent a large number of preterm deliveries. These studies would benefit by including cost-benefit analysis.

# References

Apgar, V. (1953) A proposal for a new method of evaluation of the newborn infant. *Current Researches in Anesthesia and Analgesia*, 32, 260–267.

August, R. V. (1960). Obstetric hypnoanaesthesia. *American Journal of Obstetrics and Gynecology*, 79, 1131–1138.

Barnett, E. A. (1989). *Analytical Hypnotherapy – Principles and Practice*. Glendale, CA: Westwood Pub. Co.

Bobart, V., & Brown, D. C. (2002). Medical obstetrical hypnosis and Apgar scores and the use of anaesthesia and analgesia during labor and delivery. *Hypnos*, 29(3), 132–139.

Bonica, J. J. (1963). *The Management of Pain*. Philadelphia: Lee & Febiger.

Brown, D. C., & Massarelli, E. (2002). Medical hypnosis and quadruplets: A case report. *American Journal of Clinical Hypnosis*, 45(1), 39–46.

Brown, D. C., & Murphy, M. (1999). Medical hypnosis preterm labor: A randomized clinical trial report of two pilot projects. *Hypnos*, 26(2), 77–87.

Cheek, D. B. (1995). Early use of psychotherapy in prevention of preterm labor: The application of hypnosis and ideomotor techniques with women carrying twin pregnancies. *Pre- and Perinatal Psychology Journal*, 10(1), 5–19.

Collins, M. S., & Bleyl, J. A. (1990). Seventy-one quadruplet pregnancies: Management and outcome. *American Journal of Obstetrics and Gynecology*, 162, 1384–1392.

Copper, R. L., Goldenberg, R. L., Das, A., Elder, N., Swim, M., Norman, B., et al. (1996) The preterm prediction study: Maternal stress is associated with spontaneous preterm birth at less than thirty-five weeks gestation. *American Journal of Obstetrics and Gynecology*, 175, 1286–1292.

Cyna, A. M., McAuliffe, G. L., & Andrew, M. I. (2004), Hypnosis for pain relief in labor and childbirth: A systematic review. *British Journal of Anaesthesia*, 93, 505–511.

Davidson, J. A. (1962). An assessment of the value of hypnosis in pregnancy and labor. *British Medical Journal*, 951–953.

Delee J. B. (1939). *Yearbook of Obstetrics and Gynecology*. Chicago: Yearbook Medical Publishers.

Erickson, J. C., III (1994). The use of hypnosis in anesthesia: A master class commentary. *International Journal of Clinical and Experimental Hypnosis*, 41(1), 8–12.

Flowers, C. E., et al. (1960) Pharmacologic and hypnoid analgesia effect upon labor and infant responses. *Obstetrics and Gynecology*, 16, 210–211.

Freeman R. M., Macaulay, A. J., Eve, L., & Chamberlain, G. V. P. (1986). Randomized trial of self hypnosis for analgesia in labor. *British Medical Journal*, 292, 657–659.

Goldman L. (1992). The use of hypnosis in obstetrics. *Psychiatric Medicine*, 10(4), 59–67.

Gross, H. N., & Posner, N. A. (1963). An evaluation of hypnosis for obstetric delivery. *American Journal of Obstetrics and Gynecology*, 87, 912–920.

Harmon, T. M., Hynan, M. T., & Tyre, T. E. (1990). Improved obstetric outcomes using hypnotic analgesia and skill mastery combined with childbirth education. *Journal of Consulting and Clinical Psychology*, 58(5), 525–530.

Hedegaard, M., Henriksen, T. B., Sabroe, S., & Secher, N. J. (1993). Psychological distress in pregnancy and preterm delivery. *British Medical Journal*, 307, 234–239.

Hilgard, E. R., & Hilgard, J. R. (1975). *Hypnosis and the Relief of Pain*. Los Altos, CA: William Kauffman.

Hoffman, G., & Kipenhaur, D. (1969). Medical hypnosis and its use in obstetrics. *American Journal of Medical Science*, 241, 78.

Jenkins M. W., & Pritchard, M. H. (1993). Hypnosis: Practical applications and theoretical considerations in normal labor. *British Journal of Obstetrics and Gynecology*, 100, 221–226.

Knudson, R. A. (1968). A program for improving reading efficiency through the use of suggestion. Unpublished doctoral dissertation. *Dissertation Abstracts International* 29(1-B), 359.

Kroger, W. (1977). *Clinical and Experimental Hypnosis*. Philadelphia: Lippincott.

Lederman, R. P. (1995). Relationship of anxiety, stress, and psychological development to reproductive health. *Behavioral Medicine*, 21, 101–112.

Logan, W. G. (1963). Delay of premature labor by the use of hypnosis. *American Journal of Clinical Hypnosis*, 5, 209–211.

Lou, H. C., Nordentoft, M., Jensen, F., Pryds, O., Nim, J., & Hemmingsen, R. (1992). Psychosocial stress and severe prematurity. *The Lancet*, 340, 54.

Luke, B., Mamelle, N., Keith, L., Munoz, F., Minogue, J., Papiernik, E., & Johnson, T. R. B. (1995). The association between occupational factors and preterm birth: A United States nurses study. In collaboration with the Research Committee of the Association of Women's Health, Obstetric, and Neonatal Nurses. *American Journal of Obstetrics and Gynecology*, 173, 849–862.

MacDonald, T. J., & Nathanielsz, P. W. (1991). Bilateral destruction of the fetal paraventricular nuclei prolongs gestation in sheep. *American Journal of Obstetrics and Gynecology*, 165, 764–770.

Mairs, D. A. E. (1995) Hypnosis and pain in childbirth. *Contemporary Hypnosis*, 12(2), 111–118.

Mamelle, N., Measson, A., Munoz, F., de la Bastie, A., Gerin, P., Hanauer, M. T., Collet, P., & Guyotat, J. (1989). Development and use of a self-administered questionnaire for assessment of psychologic attitudes toward pregnancy and their relation to a subsequent premature birth. *American Journal of Epidemiology*, 130(5), 989–998.

Mamelle, N., Munoz, F., Collin, D., et al. (1981). Fatigue professionale et prématurité. *Archives des Maladies Professionelles*, 42, 211–216. (Prevention of preterm labor and delivery.)

Mamelle, N., Sequeilla, M., Munoz, F., & Berland, M. (1997). Prevention of preterm birth in patients with symptoms of preterm labor: The benefits of psychologic support. *American Journal of Obstetrics and Gynecology*, l(177), 947–952.

Martin, A. (1987). The effect of hypnosis and supportive counseling on the labor processes and birth outcomes of pregnant adolescents. Doctoral dissertation: University of Florida, 1987. *Dissertation Abstracts International*, 49-08, A2114.

Martin, A. A., Schauble, P. G., Rai, S. H. J., & Curry, R. W. (2001). The effects of hypnosis on the labor processes and birth outcomes of pregnant adolescents. *Journal of Family Practice*, 50, 441–443.

Moya, F., & Jones, L. S. (1982). Medical hypnosis for obstetrics. *American Journal of Clinical. Hypnosis*, 24, 149–177.

Mutale, T., Creed, F., Maresh, M., & Hunt, L. (1991). Life events and low birthweight-analysis by infants preterm and small for gestational age. *British Journal of Obstetrics and Gynecology*, 98, 166–172.

Nathanielsz, P. W. (1992). *Life Before Birth and a Time to be Born*. Ithaca, NY: Promethean Press.

Nathanielsz, P. W. (1994). A time to be born: implications of animal studies in maternal-fetal medicine. *Birth*, 24(3), 163–169.

Newton, R. (1989). The influence of psychosocial stress in low birthweight and preterm labor. In: R. Beard, & F. Sharp Ward (Eds.). *Books on Research in Perinatal Medicine. Part III: Preterm Labor and its Consequences*, pp. 225–248.

Newton, R. W., & Hunt, L. P. (1984). Psychosocial stress in pregnancy and its relation to low birth weight. *British Medical Journal*, 288, 1191–1194.

Newton, R. W., Webster, P. A. C., Binu, P. S., Maskrey, N., & Phillips, A. B. (1979). Psychosocial stress in pregnancy and its relation to the onset of premature labor. *British Medical Journal*, 2, 411–413.

Omer, H. A. (1987). Hypnotic relaxation technique for the treatment of premature labor. *American Journal Clinical of Hypnosis*, 29, 206–213.

Oster, M. I. (1994). Psychological preparation for labor and delivery using hypnosis. *American Journal of Clinical Hypnosis*, 37(1), 12–21.

Papiernik, E., Bouyer, J., Yeaffe, K., Winisdorffer, G., Collin, D., & Dreyfus, J. (1986). Women's acceptance of a preterm birth prevention program. *American Journal of Obstetrics and Gynecology*, 155, 939–946.

Picone, T. A., Allen, L. H., Schramm, M. M., & Olsen, P. N. (1982). Pregnancy outcome in North American women: Effects of diet, cigarette smoking, and psychological stress on maternal weight gain. *American Journal of Clinical Nutrition*, 36, 1205–1213.

Roig-Garcia, S. (1961). Hypnosis in obstetrics. *American Journal of Clinical Hypnosis*, 4(1), 14–21.

Rossi, E. L. & Cheek, D. B. (1988). *Mind–Body Therapy: Methods in Ideodynamic Healing in Hypnosis*. New York: W.W. Norton.

Schwartz, M. M. (1963). The cessation of labor using hypnotic techniques. *American Journal of Clinical Hypnosis*, 5, 211–213.

Schauble, P. G., Werner, W. E. F., Rai, S. H., & Martin, A. (1998). Childbirth preparation through hypnosis: The hypnoreflexogenous protocol. *American Journal of Clinical Hypnosis*, 40(4), 273–283.

Scott, J. R., & Rose, N. B. (1976). Effect of psychoprophylaxis (Lamaze preparation) on labor and delivery in primiparas. *New England Journal of Medicine*, 294, 1205–1207.

Smith, C. A., Collins, C. T., Cyna, A. M., & Crowther, C. A. (2003). Complementary and alternative therapies for pain management in labor. *The Cochrane Database of Systematic Reviews*, 2, Art. No. CD003521. DOI: 10.1002/14651858. CD003521.

Smith, G., Egbert, L., Markowitz, R., Mosteller, F., & Beecher, H. (1966). An experimental pain method sensitive to morphine in man: The submaximum effort tourniquet technique. *Journal of Pharmacological and Experimental Therapeutics*, 154, 324–332.

Weinberg, A. (1963). Hypnosis in obstetrics and gynecology. *Clinical Obstetrics and Gynecology*, 6, 489–513.

Werner, W. (1959). Hypnosis from the viewpoint of obstetrics and clinical demonstration of the training of patients for delivery under hypnosis. *New York State Journal of Medicine*, 1561.

Werner, W. E. F., Schauble, P. G., & Knudson, M. S. (1982). An argument for the revival of hypnosis in obstetrics. *American Journal of Clinical Hypnosis*, 24, 149–171.

Williamson, H. A., Lefevre, M., & Hector, M. (1989). Association between life stresses and serious perinatal complications. *Journal of Family Practice*, 29(5), 489–496.

# *Afterword*

No longer is our highest aim to cure disease, but to prevent it.
*Sir William Osler, MD*

As mentioned in the Preface to the book, this endeavor began with the 6th Frontiers of Hypnosis Assembly held in Halifax, Nova Scotia, in 2003. That lively forum demonstrated the depth and breadth of thinking about and application of hypnosis as it is employed by diverse professionals across a range of disciplines. For one who has used it for over 40 years, it was an exciting meeting, and the seed was planted to make the work available to a larger audience. This book is offered with that purpose.

You have now had the opportunity to hear from 14 professionals, all of whom use and continue to explore this still-evolving approach. It is my hope that the contributions have added something to your own understanding of the possibilities that hypnosis encompasses, whether that understanding is in the details or in a more global sense. Each of the contributions has covered a lot of ground in a relatively limited space, and each could easily become a book in itself. Yet, taken as whole, this work presents just a glimpse of the vast potential of hypnosis, whether as an adjunct or a stand-alone approach, in almost every phase of prevention, treatment, and recovery.

When Mark Tracten suggested I put together a book from the presentations at the 6th Frontiers of Hypnosis, I got to thinking about what the goal might be.

I believe hypnosis is a much underutilized modality in clinical practice, especially in medicine. I hope this book will help to stimulate a wider use of hypnosis in practice. I have been impressed with the effects of hypnosis since one of my prenatal patients asked me to teach her to do hypnosis for the labor and delivery of her second child. She had had a prolonged, difficult, and painful forceps delivery with her first pregnancy. I suggested we discuss it at her next monthly prenatal visit. I had no training in hypnosis so I had a month to get ready. She was my first hypnosis patient. Following the usual abdominal prenatal exam at her next visit, for some reason I checked her reflexes before her first trance that day. Her ankle and knee-jerk reflexes were 2+ and 3+ before trance. Much to my surprise they were absent (zero) while in the trance! I thought, "Boy, there is something happening here, there is really something powerful going on here in trance." I had never seen this before in my medical practice. She had a much shorter labor and a spontaneous delivery of her second child and first son. She was an excellent hypnosis subject. Following that experience I offered hypnosis to all my prenatal patients, and about half of them decided to use it. At one time in rural practice I was delivering over 100 babies per year. A few years later I realized that offering hypnosis to my obstetrical patients saved me time. The women all learned self-hypnosis and received tailor-made audiotapes to reinforce the learning. Turns out, they required fewer visits and examinations during labor and delivery, and they had shorter labors, requiring fewer drugs. In a controlled study, the hypnosis babies had better Apgar scores than did the control infants.

My first book on the topic was *A System of Medical Hypnosis* by Ainsley Meares (1960). He stated that the book was intended primarily for the clinician, either in the specialized field of psychiatry or in general medicine. As a general practitioner of family medicine in those days, it met my needs. Several decades, numerous hats, and thousands of experiences later, I understand hypnosis to be both an essential and yet still somewhat misunderstood or unrecognized aspect of health delivery on every level.

When I step back, I see this volume as a prismatic presentation of clinical hypnosis for the reader to gain a more multifaceted view of it. I have had many years to enjoy such a view through my various associations: as a member of the Canadian Society of Clinical Hypnosis and the American Society of Clinical Hypnosis for over 30 years; as a founding member, in 1977, of the Clinical Hypnosis Society of Nova Scotia with Ralph Phillips, David Shieres, and others; and as a member of ASCH since my first sabbatical year in Charleston. The Canadian Federation of Hypnosis had its first organizational meeting in Halifax at the 6th Frontiers of Hypnosis in 2003.

It is important to remember that what we do in our practices with patients and clients, and what we write in journals and books about hypnosis, is very much dependent on and enriched by the perspectives forged by earlier pioneers in the field. We stand on the shoulders of many clinicians and teachers who have gone before – all of the personalities and characters that have lit up our profession through many decades. I owe a great deal to all those teachers and colleagues for their wit, wisdom, knowledge, experience and, on occasion, for their spirit and spirituality. I have had the good fortunate to meet many colorful people who have shared wonderful lessons and ideas about using hypnosis in practice.

Throughout the years, I have learned a great deal in the many stimulating workshops and scientific assemblies I have attended. Of course, I learn the most from my patients. And it is clear that context is crucial. The context in which you relate to your patient or client is central and has a bearing on the therapeutic relationship that develops over time – whether weeks, months, or years. It often comes down to what one believes is what can be accomplished. This is why I ask patients about their religion or what they believe early on and record the answer at the top of the first page of their clinical record.

Encouraging more clinicians to use hypnosis has been a slow process. Perhaps we have been working at the wrong level, waiting until school has been completed, and the postgraduate level and with practitioners.

I believe we should apply Sir William Osler's emphasis on prevention and catching folks earlier in life. We should begin introducing the value of hypnosis and self-hypnosis at a much younger age. It is always better to prevent rather than have to treat disease and illness.

I think we should adapt and apply the knowledge presented throughout this book on a more regular basis: To help patients or clients go through the investigative and treatment process…To help them cope with life problems and sickness…To reach people younger when they are in delta and theta wavelength, or the hypnogogic state…To reach them as early as 5 years old…To teach everyone to harness the ability to use hypnosis for stress prevention and to create healthier, more relaxed, and more comfortable lives.

This preventative approach could be easily and naturally incorporated into sports programs. And teachers could learn how to improve and prevent their own stress responses. Such a system could be developed as a broad-based life-learning program. Pilot projects of various types could be developed and funded by foundations, philanthropists, or others. Once people learn self-hypnosis, they can use it throughout their lives.

Each time the patient listens to an audiotape of his or her trance (made in the office), the words are the same, but the trance is different because it is heard in the context of that particular day.

William James wrote: "The greatest discovery of my generation is that human beings, by changing the inner attitudes of their minds, can change the outer aspects of their lives. It is too bad," he added, "that more people will not accept this tremendous discovery and begin living it." James died in 1910 and we still have not learned to live that insight.

## What is the Future of Hypnosis? What Do You Envision?

We have come a long way during this last century in clarifying and demonstrating how hypnosis works. We still have a lot further to go in introducing people to the practice of regular daily self-hypnosis to change the outer aspects of their lives, and in teaching them how to practice self-hypnosis to draw on that tremendous subconscious power within to change those aspects.

The first issue of the *Journal of the American Society of Clinical Hypnosis* was published the same year I did my internship training before graduating as an M.D. in 1959. Upon returning to the journal in 2008, we find the following perspectives from four articles presented in the 50th anniversary edition of the *American Journal of Clinical Hypnosis*. Each view hones in on a different aspect of hypnosis that proves essential to our contemporary understanding of its application and potential.

Mark Weisberg presents a synthesis of cultural crosscurrents. He states that hypnosis is used increasingly for health care applications in hospitals, clinics, and psychotherapy practice. He points to a substantial body of research that demonstrates the efficacy of hypnosis as part of the integrative treatment of many conditions that traditional medicine has found difficult to treat. We have come to develop more detailed expectations about the beneficial effects of hypnotic interventions for health problems. We have also come to know that in these populations hypnosis can lead not only to reduced anxiety but also to specifically altered physiological parameters.

In his article on what we can do with hypnosis, David Wark summarizes the search for efficacious hypnotic treatments. Eighteen major meta-analyses were reviewed and the results evaluated using the criteria of Chambless and Hollon (1998). The analysis identified 32 disorders for which hypnosis can be considered a possible treatment, five for which it seems effective, and two for which it appears specific.

Jeffrey Zeig represents hypnosis as a "dramatic process of psychotherapy." He explains that psychotherapy can be conceived as a symbolic drama in which patients can experientially realize their capacity to change. Methods derived from hypnosis can empower therapy without the use of formal trance. A case conducted by Milton Erickson is presented and deconstructed in order to reveal Erickson's therapeutic patterns. A model is offered for adding drama to therapy, and the model is placed into a larger model of choice points in psychotherapy.

Howard Sutcher discusses hypnosis and how it has reached its current status in medicine, psychiatry, psychology, and dentistry. The mechanisms underlying hypnosis and how hypnosis differs from other cognitive states are almost totally unknown. With the exceptions of suggestions for pain control, current concepts of high, medium, low, or non-hypnotizability do not reliably predict clinical outcomes for most medical, psychiatric, or dental disorders. Four case studies, representative of many others, chosen retrospectively from a practice that spans 45 years, illustrate how traditional or modern hypnotizability assessment is irrelevant in the clinical setting. Although the four patients differed obviously and vastly in hypnotizability, they all benefited from the use of hypnosis.

How is all of this related to private practice? The lessons based on two common habits that were part of my family practice help clarify the importance of hypnosis as an integral aspect of supporting well-being.

I used to do routine microscopic urinalysis on all children seen in my family practice. At a certain point, a colleague and I did a retrospective study on all the children I had seen during my last year of private practice. Kwang Yang, a family medicine resident, did the research work and I provided the patient charts and hospital records (see Brown & Yang, 1972). In that one year, 102 cases of childhood urinary-tract infection (UTI) were detected and treated.

A specimen of "clean" mid-stream urine was collected from each of the 690 patients under the age of 15 years old seen from June 1, 1967 to May 31, 1968. The urine was tested routinely and examined microscopically, and it was cultured in cases of recurrent UTI. Routine urinalysis and the physician's alertness are essential to diagnose and treat UTI in its early stages in children, and thus prevent renal disease in later life.

Another interest of mine was prevention of invasive carcinoma of the cervix through routine pap smears. There are very few screening agents or tests that have a cost-benefit factor of seven to one: that is, for every dollar expense of the test, seven dollars are saved in the cost of therapy, including advanced disease and even death (Brown, 1966, 1967, 1968, 1969, 1976, 1979, 1980, 1990, 1998). No woman should die from cancer of the cervix. Women who have a pap smear and proper follow-up done each year don't.

Just as we do screening tests, histories, and physical examinations to diagnose and treat physical disease early for improved results and prognosis, we can do screening tests and histories for early diagnosis and management of emotional and mental illnesses for improved outcome and improved quality of life.

The most common of these illnesses are anxiety, depression, and insomnia. Many people with chronic pain may present to the practitioner as depression or insomnia. Every person will reflect a slightly different mixture or combination of issues – and common problems can manifest in many different ways.

There are two easy self-administered anxiety and depression rating scales. They can be used as screening tests to be filled in while patients and clients are in the waiting room. They also may be used as a means of measuring progress and response to therapy over the years. The Zung Self-Rated Depression Scale can be employed to diagnose depression and follow response to treatment and management. The Hamilton Anxiety Scale may also be used to evaluate progress in therapy and monitor the severity of anxiety or assist in its management.

In the field of hypnosis clinicians continue to pose many of the most interesting and complex questions (Fromm & Nash, 1992). It is my hope that some of the clinicians reading this book will go back and look closely at their practices to develop a question – a research question in their area of a special interest. Perhaps this cutting-edge question will expand our knowledge in an important area of therapy or prevention. Perhaps the question will be pursued alongside other disciplines and together this research team will find an answer that helps improve peace of mind, support achievement, and foster a sense of self-mastery that emphasizes quality of life.

The words of Wilder Penfield, former chief neurosurgeon at the Montreal Neurological Institute, are particularly apt when I think about our task:

> To gather knowledge and to find out new knowledge is the noblest occupation of the physician. To apply that knowledge with sympathy born of understanding, to the relief of human suffering, is his loveliest occupation.
> *E. W. Archibald (1872–1945)*

# *References*

Archibald, E. W. (2008). The Square Knot. Department of Surgery Newsletter, McGill.

Bobart, V., & Brown, D. C. (2002). Medical obstetrical hypnosis and Apgar scores and the use of anaesthesia and analgesia during labor and delivery. *Hypnos*, XXIX(3): 132–139.

Brown, D. C. (1965). My first dozen: Twelve cases of carcinoma in situ of cervix. *Nova Scotia Medical Bulletin*, April.

Brown, D. C. (1966). Early diagnosis of carcinoma of the cervix in general practice. *College of General Practice of Canada Journal*, 12: 30–4.

Brown, D. C. (1967/68). What 2630 pap smears taught me. *Consultant* (US), November/December; *Consultant* (Canadian), March/April.

Brown, D. C. (1969). Positive smear. *Canadian Family Physician*, 15(6).

Brown, D. C. (1976). Early detection of cancer in women. Editoral introduction to a brief symposium. *Primary Care*, 3(3).

Brown, D. C. (1979). Cancer of the cervix: A twenty year follow-up. *Canadian Family Physician*, 25: 1032–1039.

Brown, D. C. (1980). The pap smear: Annual or not? – Dr. Brown replies. *Canadian Family Physician*, 25: 183–184.

Brown, D. C. (1983). Stress and the physician. A preventive approach: Editorial. *Canadian Family Physician*, 29: 396–398.

Brown, D. C. (1990). Pap screening in the over 60 year old female. *Nova Scotia Medical Journal*, 69: 191–3 and 182.

Brown, D. C. (1998). A group hypnosis smoking cessation program: Six month follow-up. *Hypnos*, 25(2): 98–103.

Brown, D. C. (1999). Medical hypnosis and preterm labor. A randomized clinical trial. Report of two pilot projects. *Hypnos*, 26(2): 77–87.

Brown, D. C. & Murphy, M. (1997). Medical hypnosis and plasma prostaglandins in preterm labor: Report of a pilot project. Workshop presentation by D. C. Brown at the 14th International Congress of Hypnosis. San Diego, CA.

Brown, D. C. & Yang, K. (1972). Childhood urinary tract infections in family practice. *Canadian Family Physician*, 18: 39–42.

Chambless, D. L., & Hollon, S. D. (1988). Defining empirically supported therapies. *Journal of Consulting and Clinical Psychology*, 66(1): 7–18.

Crawford, H. J., Knebel, T., Kaplan, L., Vendema, J. M., Xie, M., Jamison, S., & Pribram, K. H. (1998). Hypnotic analgesia: 1. Somotosensory event related potential changes to noxious stimuli, and 2. Transfer learning to reduce chronic low back pain. *International Journal of Clinical Experimental Hypnosis*, 46(1): 92–132.

Douglas, K. (2008). *Newsweek*, August 11, p. 20.

Fromm, E., & Nash, M. R. (1992). *Contemporary Hypnosis Research*. New York: Guilford.

Hamilton, M. (1959). The assessment of anxiety states by rating. *British Journal of Medical Psychology*, 32: 50–55.

Havens, R. A., & Walters, C. (1989). *Hypnotherapy Scripts – a Neo-Ericksonian Approach to Persuasive Healing*. New York: Brunner/Mazel.

James, W. (1893). *The Principles of Psychology*. New York: Henry Holt.

Meares, A. (1960). *A System of Medical Hypnosis*. Philadelphia: W.B. Saunders.

Penfield, W. (1963). *The Second Career*. Boston: Little Brown.

Pert, C. (1997). The physiology of emotion and mind/body communication. Plenary Presentation at 14th International Congress of Hypnosis, San Diego, CA.

Pribram, K. H. (1997). Dissociation as a function of the deep and surface structure of memory. Plenary Presentation at 15th International Congress of Hypnosis, San Diego, CA.

Rossi, E. L. & Ryan, M. O. (Eds.) (1992). *The Seminars, Workshops and Lectures of Milton H. Erickson. Vol I: Healing in Hypnosis; Vol II: Life Reframing in Hypnosis; Vol III: Mind-Body Communication in Hypnosis; Vol. IV: Creative Choice in Hypnosis*. New York: Irvington.

Sabourin, M. E., Cutcomb, S. D., Crawford, H. J., & Prebram, K. (1990). EEG correlates of hypnotic susceptibility and hypnotic trance: Special analysis and coherence. *International Journal of Psychophysiology*, 10(2): 125–142.

Sutcher, H. (2008). Hypnosis, hypnotizability and treatment. *American Journal of Clinical Hypnosis*, 51(1): 57–67.

Wark, D. M. (2008). What we can do with hypnosis: A brief note. *American Journal of Clinical Hypnosis*, 51(1): 29–36.

Weisberg, M. B. (2008). 50 years of hypnosis in medicine and clinical health psychology: A synthesis of cultural crosscurrents. *American Journal of Clinical Hypnosis*, 51(1): 13–27.

Zeig, J. K. (2008). The (dramatic) process of psychotherapy. *American Journal of Clinical Hypnosis*, 51(1): 41–55.

Zung, W. W. (1965). A self-rating depression scale. *Archives of General Psychiatry*, 12: 63–70.

## Further Resources

http://www.anxiety help.org/information/hama.html
http://www.medalreq.com/qhc/medal/ch18/18_04/18-04-03-ver9.php3
http://www.depression-webworld.homa/hama_print1.htm
http://www.psychiatrictimes.com/clinical-scales
http://www.depression-help-resource.com/depression-test.htm
http://www.healthnet.umassmed.edu/mhealth/ZungSelfRatedDepressionScale.pdf

# *About the Editor*

Donald Corey Brown, BSc, MD, CCFP, FCFP, ABFP, is an approved consultant in medical hypnosis by the American Society of Clinical Hypnosis.

Following numerous years of rural family practice, Dr. Brown was appointed Director of Dalhousie University Residency Program in Family Practice, and went on to become Founding Director, Department of Family Medicine, Dalhousie University Medical School. A respected lecturer and researcher, he has presented workshops, seminars, and scientific exhibits throughout Canada, the United States, Switzerland, Mexico, Hong Kong, and Australia. He is licensed to practice family medicine and medical hypnosis therapy in Nova Scotia.

Dr. Brown has been a member and/or has chaired countless regional and national committees and boards, including serving as Chair of the editorial advisory board for *Canadian Family Physician*. Among his many other undertakings, he was an editorial consultant and a member of the editorial board for the launching of *Primary Care Clinics of North America*.

Now retired from his position as Associate Professor, Dalhousie University Medical School (1996), Dr. Brown is currently involved in full-time private practice as a consultant in medical hypnosis.

# Index